Thymoma

Guest Editor

FEDERICO VENUTA, MD

THORACIC
SURGERY CLINICS

www.thoracic.theclinics.com

Consulting Editor

MARK K. FERGUSON, MD

February 2011 • Volume 21 • Number 1

SAUNDERS an imprint of ELSEVIER, Inc.

W.B. SAUNDERS COMPANY
A Division of Elsevier Inc.

1600 John F. Kennedy Boulevard ● Suite 1800 ● Philadelphia, Pennsylvania 19103-2899

http://www.theclinics.com

THORACIC SURGERY CLINICS Volume 21, Number 1
February 2011 ISSN 1547-4127, ISBN-13: 978-1-4557-0513-9

Editor: Ruth Malwitz
Developmental Editor: Donald Mumford

Thoracic Surgery Clinics (ISSN 1547-4127) is published quarterly by Elsevier Inc., 360 Park Avenue South, New York, NY 10010-1710. Months of publication are February, May, August, and November. Business and editorial offices: 1600 John F. Kennedy Boulevard, Suite 1800, Philadelphia, PA 19103-2899. Periodicals postage paid at New York, NY, and additional mailing offices. Subscription prices are $295.00 per year (US individuals), $385.00 per year (US institutions), $141.00 per year (US Students), $367.00 per year (Canadian individuals), $487.00 per year (Canadian institutions), $192.00 per year (Canadian and foreign students), $391.00 per year (foreign individuals), and $487.00 per year (foreign institutions). Foreign air speed delivery is included in all Clinics' subscription prices. All prices are subject to change without notice. **POSTMASTER:** Send address changes to Thoracic Surgery Clinics, Elsevier Health Sciences Division, Subscription Customer Service, 3251 Riverport Lane, Maryland Heights, MO 63043. **Customer Service (orders, claims, online, change of address): Telephone: 1-800-654-2452 (U.S. and Canada); 314-447-8871 (outside U.S. and Canada). Fax: 314-447-8029. Email: journalscustomerservice-usa@elsevier.com (for print support); journalsonlinesupport-usa@elsevier.com (for online support).**

Reprints. For copies of 100 or more, of articles in this publication, please contact Commercial Rights Department, Elsevier Inc., 360 Park Avenue South, New York, NY 10010-1710. Tel: (212) 633-3812; Fax: (212) 462-1935; E-mail: reprints@elsevier.com.

Thoracic Surgery Clinics is covered in *MEDLINE/PubMed (Index Medicus)* and *EMBASE/Excerpta Medica*.

Printed and bound by CPI Group (UK) Ltd, Croydon, CR0 4YY

Transferred to Digital Print 2012

Contributors

CONSULTING EDITOR

MARK K. FERGUSON, MD
Professor of Surgery, Section of Cardiac and
Thoracic Surgery, The University of Chicago
Medical Center, Chicago, Illinois

GUEST EDITOR

FEDERICO VENUTA, MD
Department of Thoracic Surgery, Policlinico
Umberto I, University of Rome Sapienza,
Cattedra di Chirurgia Toracica, Rome, Italy

AUTHORS

PAOLA CAMPISI, MD
Attending Physician, Division of Pathology,
University of Torino, Corso Bramante, Torino,
Italy

FRANK C. DETTERBECK, MD
Professor and Chief, Section of Thoracic
Surgery, Yale University School of Medicine,
New Haven, Connecticut

PIER LUIGI FILOSSO, MD
Assistant Professor, Division of Thoracic
Surgery, University of Torino, Via Genova,
Torino, Italy

YOSHITAKA FUJII, MD, PhD
Professor, Department of Surgery II, Nagoya
City University Medical School, Mizuhoku,
Nagoya, Japan

GIUSEPPE GIACCONE, MD, PhD
Chief, Medical Oncology Branch, National
Cancer Institute, National Institutes of Health,
Bethesda, Maryland

NICOLAS GIRARD, MD
Radiotherapy Department, Lyon-Sud Hospital,
Pierre-Bénite; Department of Respiratory
Medicine, Pilot Unit for the Management of
Rare Intrathoracic Tumors, Louis Pradel
Hospital; Claude Bernard University, Lyon,
France

KEMP H. KERNSTINE, MD, PhD
Director, Lung Cancer and Thoracic Oncology
Program, City of Hope National Medical
Center, Duarte, California

WALTER KLEPETKO, MD
Department of Cardiothoracic Surgery, Vienna
Medical University, Vienna, Austria

FLORIAN LÄNGER, MD
Professor, Thoracic Surgery, Institute
of Pathology, Medizinische Hochschule
Hannover, Hannover, Germany

KARL K. LIMMER, MD
Department of Surgery, University of California
San Diego School of Medicine, San Diego,
California

ALEXANDER MARX, MD
Professor, Institute of Pathology, University
Medical Center Mannheim, University of
Heidelberg, Mannheim, Germany

MIRELLA MARINO, MD
Department of Pathology, Regina Elena
National Cancer Institute, Rome, Italy

FRANÇOISE MORNEX, MD, PhD
Radiotherapy Department, Lyon-Sud Hospital,
Pierre-Bénite; Claude Bernard University,
Lyon, France

DOMENICO NOVERO, MD
Attending Physician, Division of Pathology,
University of Torino, Corso Bramante, Torino,
Italy

ALBERTO OLIARO, MD
Professor of Thoracic Surgery, Head of the
Division of Thoracic Surgery, University of
Torino, Via Genova, Torino, Italy

ALDEN M. PARSONS, MD
Thoracic Surgery, Rex Thoracic Specialists,
Raleigh, North Carolina

MAURO PIANTELLI, MD
Professor of Pathology, Department
of Oncology and Neurosciences,
"G. D'Annunzio" University and Foundation
Chieti-Pescara, Chieti, Italy

ARUN RAJAN, MD
Staff Clinician, Medical Oncology Branch,
National Cancer Institute, National Institutes
of Health, Bethesda, Maryland

ERINO A. RENDINA, MD
Department of Thoracic Surgery, Ospedale
Sant'Andrea, University of Rome Sapienza,
Rome, Italy

RALF RIEKER, MD
Professor, Institute for Pathology, University
Hospital, Erlangen; Institute for Pathology,
University Hospital, Heidelberg, Germany

GAETANO ROCCO, MD
Pascale Foundation, National Cancer Institute,
Naples, Italy

ENRICO RUFFINI, MD
Associate Professor, Division of Thoracic
Surgery, University of Torino, Via Genova,
Torino, Italy

PHILIPP STRÖBEL, MD
Professor, Institute of Pathology, University
Medical Center Mannheim, University of
Heidelberg, Mannheim, Germany

PASCAL A. THOMAS, MD
Professor of Thoracic Surgery, Department
of Thoracic Surgery, University Hospitals of
Marseille, University of the Mediterranean,
and North University Hospital, Chemin des
Bourrely, Marseille, France

ALPER TOKER, MD
Professor, Thoracic Surgery, Istanbul
University, Turkey

NORIYUKI TOMIYAMA, MD, PhD
Professor and Chairman, Department of
Radiology, Osaka University Graduate School
of Medicine, Osaka, Japan

FEDERICO VENUTA, MD
Department of Thoracic Surgery, Policlinico
Umberto I, University of Rome Sapienza,
Cattedra di Chirurgia Toracica, Rome, Italy

CAMERON D. WRIGHT, MD
Professor of Surgery, Division of Thoracic
Surgery, Massachusetts General Hospital,
Harvard Medical School, Boston,
Massachusetts

MASAHIRO YANAGAWA, MD, PhD
Attending Staff, Department of Radiology,
Osaka University Graduate School
of Medicine, Osaka, Japan

MARCIN ZIELIŃSKI, MD, PhD
Head of Department of Thoracic Surgery,
Pulmonary Hospital, Zakopane, Poland

Contents

Thymic epithelial tumors, such as thymomas and thymic carcinomas, are the most common primary neoplasms of the mediastinum. In 1999, the World Health Organization (WHO) proposed a consensus classification of thymic epithelial tumors based on the morphology of the epithelial cells and the ratio of lymphocytes to epithelial cells, which was revised in 2004. The latest classification system stratifies thymic epithelial tumors into six categories: types A, AB, B1, B2, B3, and thymic carcinoma. This article describes the prediction of thymoma histology and stage on the basis of radiographic criteria by reviewing the following: the WHO histologic classification of thymic epithelial tumors, the clinical staging of thymomas based on prognosis, and the radiographic appearance of thymomas according to the WHO histologic classification.

Neuroendocrine tumors of the thymus (NETTs) are unusual thymic neoplasms that were misdiagnosed as thymomas until the 1970s, when they eventually acquired a distinct identity. No collective large series have been published so far, and information about clinical presentation, diagnosis, histology, and treatment is derived from analysis of the case series and case reports published over a long period. NETTs are more aggressive than their pulmonary and abdominal counterparts, presenting at a more advanced stage, often with distant metastases, and are associated with poor long-term survival. Most patients are symptomatic at presentation as a result of the local invasion. Twenty percent to 30% of the cases are associated with endocrine disorders, mostly Cushing syndrome and multiple endocrine neoplasia syndrome. There is no official staging system for these tumors and investigators rely on the Masaoka staging system used for thymomas. Histologically, 2 classification are used: the World Health Organization and the Armed Forces Institute of Pathology classifications. Histologically, most tumors show moderately to poorly differentiated histologic features, reflecting their aggressive clinical behavior. Surgery is the most effective treatment option, although the aggressiveness of the tumor often requires extensive resection. Chemotherapy and radiotherapy may be used either preoperatively or postoperatively, although the small number of patients does not allow the design of standard guidelines about optimal schedules and doses. Survival depends on stage at presentation, histologic degree of differentiation, associated endocrine syndromes, and resectability rate. Recurrences are frequent after surgery and may be locoregional or distant. Surgery is recommended when feasible in the treatment of locoregional recurrences.

The second edition of the World Health Organization (WHO) classification of thymic tumors (2004) has resumed the previous separation of thymic carcinomas (TCs) from thymomas. This "reseparation" was mainly based on new genetic data.

Consequently, it is no longer recommended to label TCs as type C thymomas. TCs are very heterogeneous and comprise squamous, basaloid cell, mucoepidermoid, neuroendocrine, and many other subtypes. They resemble morphologic mimics in other organs and are labeled accordingly. However, only thymic squamous cell carcinomas (TSCCs) and lymphoepithelioma-like carcinomas are relatively common. For TSCCs, quite specific immunohistochemical markers (eg, CD5, CD70, CD117, CD205, FOXN1) and chromosomal gains and losses have been defined that help to distinguish TSCCs not only from malignant thymomas but also from pulmonary squamous cell carcinomas. Recognition of these differences is clinically important, because the prognosis of TSCC is better compared with the other TC subtypes and also compared with lung tumors. Considering the need to treat advanced TC more effectively, disparate findings in predictive molecular markers (eg, KIT mutations in TSCC, but not in thymomas) suggest that targeted treatments will have to be different in thymomas and TC. Preliminary data from single case collections and small treatment trials support this prediction.

Immunohistochemistry of Thymic Epithelial Tumors as a Tool in Translational Research 33

Mirella Marino and Mauro Piantelli

Due to their heterogeneity and infrequency, thymic epithelial cell tumors (TET) represent a diagnostic as well as a therapeutic problem. In the early stage of disease TET are usually cured by performing radical resections, whereas in advanced stages of disease they are usually radically unresectable from the beginning, and often show multiple relapses and/or intra- or extrathoracic metastases. Trained pathologists are required in TET diagnostics; awareness of the complexity of the mediastinum and of the differential diagnostic possibilities is mandatory. Immunohistochemical (IHC) studies play a fundamental role in oncologic surgical pathology. Among the many uses of IHC in cancer research, studies on a possible association between biomarker expression and treatment outcomes dominate the clinical translational research applications. This article reports on and discusses the role of IHC in diagnostic and translational research of TET.

Management of Myasthenic Patients with Thymoma 47

Marcin Zieliński

Myasthenia gravis (MG) associated with thymomas differs from nonthymomatous MG, and thymomas associated with MG are also different from non-MG thymomas. According to the World Health Organization classification, the incidence of MG in thymomas was the highest in the subtypes B2, B1, and AB. Transsternal approach is still regarded as the gold standard for surgical treatment of thymomas. Less-invasive techniques of thymectomy are promising, but it is too early to estimate their real oncological value. In the series including more than 100 patients, the prognosis for survival is better in patients with thymomas associated with MG than in those with non-MG thymomas, and the prognosis for patients with MG associated with thymoma is worse than that for patients with nonthymomatous MG.

Management of Stage I and II Thymoma 59

Frank C. Detterbeck and Alden M. Parsons

With a knowledgeable assessment of the clinical presentation and demographic and radiologic characteristics, most thymomas can be reliably identified preoperatively without the need for a biopsy. Surgery is the mainstay of treatment for stage I and II thymoma. The rate of complete resection is essentially 100% by open techniques, and recurrences are rare. A complete thymectomy via a sternotomy is the standard approach. Adjuvant radiotherapy after a complete resection does not appear to be of benefit. In the rare event of a recurrence, an aggressive approach should be taken with re-resection whenever possible.

Minimally Invasive and Robotic-Assisted Thymus Resection

Karl K. Limmer and Kemp H. Kernstine

Thymectomy for thymoma has traditionally been performed through a transsternal approach because of the excellent exposure that that the median sternotomy provides. Minimally invasive alternatives, such as transcervical thymectomy, video-assisted thymectomy, and robotic thymectomy, have not been extensively evaluated for this disease process. It is uncertain which patients may benefit from minimally invasive approaches and data regarding the oncologic effectiveness of these techniques remains to be established. However, given the excellent capability of these techniques to perform a complete and extensive thymectomy, there does appear to be a role for minimally invasive thymectomy in the treatment of thymoma.

Surgical Management of Stage III Thymic Tumors

Federico Venuta, Erino A. Rendina, Walter Klepetko, and Gaetano Rocco

Thymic tumors are classified as stage III when they clearly invade the surrounding structures: pericardium, great vessels (superior vena cava, innominate veins, ascending aorta, and main pulmonary artery), lung parenchyma, phrenic nerves, and chest wall. Surgical treatment with or without induction therapy should always aim to complete resection removing en bloc all the involved structures. Also, extended procedures are justified because only R0 resection allows long-term survival.

Stage IVA Thymoma: Patterns of Spread and Surgical Management

Cameron D. Wright

Stage IVA disease can be de novo disease or more commonly represent recurrent disease. The pleura is the most common site of relapse after thymoma resection. Local pleural disease is usually simply resected. This is usually combined with either induction or adjuvant chemotherapy. The ultimate extended surgery for advanced thymic tumors is an extrapleural pneumonectomy done for extensive pleural disease. This rarely performed operation is done for both stage IVA disease found at initial presentation and for recurrent disease as a salvage procedure. Again, these advanced patients with pleural spread are probably best managed by induction chemotherapy followed by resection.

The Role of Radiotherapy in the Management of Thymic Tumors

Nicolas Girard and Françoise Mornex

Radiotherapy is a major therapeutic modality for thymic malignancies. The exact role of adjuvant radiotherapy after complete resection is still debated for stage II through III tumors. Histology or size, capsular invasion, and even molecular data may be included in the decision making. Radiotherapy may be recommended for stage III thymomas, thymic carcinoma, or after incomplete surgical resection. Combination with chemotherapy may be useful, and must be further evaluated using validated end points, including 5- and 10-year time-to-progression and overall survival. Several initiatives have been taken worldwide to launch collaborative studies in the field, including prospective trials specifically readdressing the role of radiotherapy for thymic malignancies.

> Although thymoma and thymic carcinoma are rare malignancies, they constitute a large proportion of tumors of the anterior mediastinum. Surgery forms the mainstay of therapy; however, thymic malignancies are sensitive to chemotherapy and radiation therapy also. Systemic chemotherapy is primarily used for treatment of metastatic or recurrent disease. Chemotherapy is also used as a component of multimodality treatment in the neoadjuvant setting with the aim of increasing the chances of achieving a complete surgical resection. In this article we outline various clinical trials that have been performed to evaluate the role of chemotherapy in the treatment of thymic malignancies.

> Significant efforts have been made to dissect the molecular pathways involved in the carcinogenesis of thymic malignancies. Research is hampered by the rarity of the tumor, controversies about histopathologic classification, and the lack of established cell lines and animal models. Insights into the biology of these tumors have been made following anecdotal clinical responses to targeted therapies. This article reviews current knowledge about the molecular data that define molecular subsets and support the use of targeted therapies in thymic tumors.

> Guidelines for treatment of thymoma are prevalent in US literature, and many have been published by organizations in the United Kingdom, Canada, and Japan. This article reviews these many guidelines and summarizes them for the reader.

> Thymic epithelial tumors (TETs) are rare thoracic malignancies, with an overall incidence of 1.5 per million people. The TET Registry Project aims at federating an international network to provide a resource to support studies on the epidemiology and clinical management and monitoring some standards of clinical care of these tumors. Recorded data span all the specifications of the management of TET: paraneoplastic syndromes, histologic subtypes, diagnostic and staging issues, multimodal treatment strategies, and exceptional surgeries and therapies. Data collection for the registry is done both prospectively and retrospectively through different paths to allow the involvement of as many centers as possible, including data-sharing arrangements with some already established databases. This ambitious project implies the early setting of strong quality assurance measures looking at completeness, consistency, and accuracy of the data. These measures require a significant and long-term financial support that will also be free of possible sources of conflicts of interests.

Thoracic Surgery Clinics

RELATED INTEREST

Hematology/Oncology Clinics of North America Volume 22, Issue 3 (June 2008)
Thymic Epithelial Neoplasms: A Comprehensive Review of Diagnosis and Treatment
Cesar A. Moran and Saul Suster, *Guest Editors*

THE CLINICS ARE NOW AVAILABLE ONLINE!

Access your subscription at:
www.theclinics.com

Preface

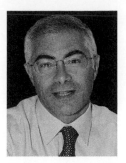

Federico Venuta, MD
Guest Editor

Epithelial thymic tumors are still a controversial subject sparking continuous debate in the international literature. Lack of agreement persists about the clinical impact of the WHO classification, the staging system, and multidisciplinary management. This clearly contributes to a rise in interest regarding thymoma and thymic carcinoma, including the efforts of thoracic surgeons, pathologists, immunologists, and medical and radiation oncologists. However, answers will not be available until we understand the biology, pathology, and clinical behavior of these tumors. For this reason a closer cooperation with basic scientists should be pursued.

The European Society of Thoracic Surgeons (ESTS) gathered a number of experts into a group (the ESTS Thymic Working Group) to work on this project. This issue of the *Thoracic Surgery Clinics* is the first tangible result of this process, providing an overview of the "state of the art" on thymic tumors. Henceforth, increased cooperation between dedicated experts, working groups, and associations hopefully will lead to the development of uniform guidelines for managing thymoma patients.

I would like to address my special thanks to my colleagues in the steering committee of the ESTS Thymic Working Group, Frank Detterbeck, Pascal Thomas, Gaetano Rocco, and Enrico Ruffini, who participated with enthusiasm to this project and strongly contributed to develop a list of interesting articles covering most of the debated topics in this field. I would also extend my personal thanks to all the members of the group who participated with their work and expertise to the preparation of the articles. We have also involved several authors external to the group; their help has strongly contributed to improve the quality of this *Thoracic Surgery Clinics* issue.

A special thank goes to Mark Ferguson, consulting editor and great friend, for his enthusiasm and support; without his continuous help it would have been impossible to achieve this goal.

Finally, a special thank goes to Saunders and to the editorial staff, in particular, Mrs Catherine Bewick and Mrs Ruth Malwitz; their continuous support greatly facilitated our work.

Federico Venuta, MD
The European Society of Thoracic Surgery
Thymic Working Group

Head Lung Transplantation Program
Department of Thoracic Surgery
University of Rome Sapienza
Policlinico Umberto I
Rome, Italy

E-mail address:
federico.venuta@uniroma1.it

EUROPEAN SOCIETY OF THORACIC SURGEONS (ESTS) THYMIC WORKING GROUP

Steering Committee

Frank Detterbeck (USA)
Pascal Thomas (France)
Gaetano Rocco (Italy)
Enrico Ruffini (Italy)
Federico Venuta (Italy)

Members of the Group

M. Zielinski (Poland): surgery in patients with MG
E. Ruffini (Italy): treatment of recurrence
W. Klepetko (Austria): extended resections
M. Marino (Italy), A. Marx and P. Stroebel (Germany): pathology
G. Giaccone (USA), M. Hatton (GB), P. Loehrer (USA): oncology
F. Mornex (France): radiation therapy
N. Girard (France): targeted therapy
A. Evoli (Italy): neurology

Thorac Surg Clin 21 (2011) xi
doi:10.1016/j.thorsurg.2010.09.003
1547-4127/11/$ — see front matter © 2011 Elsevier Inc. All rights reserved.

Prediction of Thymoma Histology and Stage by Radiographic Criteria

Masahiro Yanagawa, MD, PhD,
Noriyuki Tomiyama, MD, PhD*

KEYWORDS

- World Health Organization classification
- Thymic epithelial tumors • Computed tomography
- Magnetic resonance imaging
- Positron emission tomography

Thymic epithelial tumors, such as thymomas and thymic carcinomas, are the most common primary neoplasms of the mediastinum. Because there are variable morphologic appearances in these tumors, many studies have been performed for evaluating the correlation between morphologic characteristics and clinical behavior. In 1999, the World Health Organization (WHO) proposed a consensus classification of thymic epithelial tumors based on the morphology of the epithelial cells and the ratio of lymphocytes to epithelial cells,[1] which was then revised in 2004 by adding some recently recognized entities together with updated diagnostic criteria.[2] The latest classification system stratifies thymic epithelial tumors into 6 categories: types A, AB, B1, B2, B3, and thymic carcinoma. The clinical features of thymic epithelial tumors are reflected in the WHO histologic classification, which may contribute to the clinical assessment and treatment of patients with thymoma.[3–6] Diagnostic imaging is important for such clinical assessment and treatment. The computed tomography (CT) and magnetic resonance imaging (MRI) findings of thymic epithelial tumors classified according to the WHO histologic classification have been mentioned in previous reports.[7–9] However, we must recognize that there are limits in differentiating the various histologic subtypes by only radiographic criteria.

This article describes the prediction of thymoma histology and stage by radiographic criteria by reviewing the following: the WHO histologic classification of thymic epithelial tumors, the clinical staging of thymomas based on prognosis, and the radiographic appearance of thymomas according to the WHO histologic classification.

WHO HISTOLOGIC CLASSIFICATION OF THYMIC EPITHELIAL TUMORS

A thymoma is defined as a neoplasm arising from thymic epithelial cells. The WHO histologic classification of thymic epithelial tumors was originally presented in 1999[1] and later modified in 2004.[2] In the initial WHO classification system proposed in 1999, thymic epithelial tumors were classified into 6 categories: types A, AB, B1, B2, B3, and C. All kinds of thymic carcinomas were defined as type C thymomas. However, the category classification type C thymoma was eliminated from the system in the 2004 revision because type C thymoma showed a morphologic characterization resembling malignant neoplasms arising from other organs besides the thymus. At present, in the revised WHO classification system, thymomas are classified into 5 types (types A, AB, B1, B2, and B3) according to the morphology and atypia of the neoplastic epithelial cells and the abundance of nonneoplastic lymphocytes, and thymic

Department of Radiology, Osaka University Graduate School of Medicine, 2-2 Yamadaoka, Suita-city, Osaka, 565-0871, Japan
* Corresponding author.
E-mail address: tomiyama@radiol.med.osaka-u.ac.jp

Thorac Surg Clin 21 (2011) 1–12
doi:10.1016/j.thorsurg.2010.08.008
1547-4127/11/$ – see front matter © 2011 Elsevier Inc. All rights reserved.

carcinomas are designated as all nonorganotypic malignant epithelial neoplasms other than germ cell tumors. Although we spare detailed explanations in this article, rare thymomas unable to be categorized under that system are as follows: micronodular thymoma with lymphoid stroma, metaplastic thymoma, microscopic thymoma, sclerosing thymoma, and lipofibroadenoma.[10-14]

Thymomas are mainly divided into 2 groups (types A and B) depending on morphology of the neoplastic epithelial cells and their nuclei: type A is defined as thymomas with neoplastic spindle-shaped epithelial cells and type B is defined as thymomas with neoplastic epithelial cells in a dendritic or epithelioid shape. Thymomas with both type A and type B components are defined as type AB. Type B thymomas are further divided into 3 subtypes (B1, B2, and B3) according to the abundance of lymphocytes and the emergence of atypical neoplastic cells. Atypia of neoplastic epithelial cells increases in the order of type B1, B2, and B3: type B1 has a cortex mimicking a normal thymus with a large number of lymphocytes; type B2 is a cortical thymoma with less infiltration of lymphocytes than type B1; and type B3 is predominantly composed of epithelial cells having a round or polygonal shape and exhibiting no or mild atypia, admixed with a minor component of lymphocytes. The WHO histologic classification system is summarized in **Table 1**. The WHO classification reflects the clinical features of these tumors and correlates with prognosis. Type B2 and B3 thymomas (high-risk group) are more malignant than types A, AB, and B1 (low-risk group) in terms of invasiveness, postoperative survival, and tumor recurrence.[3,15] Patients with type A, AB, and B1 thymomas can be primarily treated by surgical resection, whereas patients with type B2 and B3 thymomas sometimes require preoperative induction chemotherapy or radiation therapy.[16]

CLINICAL STAGING OF THYMOMAS BY POSTOPERATIVE SURVIVAL

There have been many studies about the prognoses of patients with thymomas. The Masaoka and colleagues[17] staging system, which is based on invasion to the surrounding organs such as pleura, pericardia, great vessels, and lung tissues, is generally accepted as the most valuable prognostic factor. This clinical staging is useful for predicting the postoperative survival of patients with thymomas.[17-26] The Masaoka staging system is as follows (**Table 2**): stage I, encapsulated tumor without microscopic evidence of capsular invasion; stage II, microscopic or macroscopic invasion of the surrounding fatty tissue or the mediastinal pleura; stage III, macroscopic invasion of neighboring organs, such as the pericardium, great vessels, or lung; and stage IV, pericardial or pleural dissemination (IVa) and lymph node or distant metastases (IVb). Regarding survival rates according to the Masaoka staging system (see **Table 2**), the 5-year survival rates[17] were 96% for patients with stage I disease, 86% for patients with stage II disease, 69% for patients with stage III disease, and 50% for patients with stage IV disease. The 20-year survival rates[3] were 89% for patients with stage I disease, 91% for patients with stage II disease, and 49% for patients with stage III disease. No patient with stage IVa or IVb disease survived for more than 20 years. Thus, thymomas have a more indolent nature than other malignant tumors.

On the other hand, several investigators have confirmed a significant correlation between the WHO histologic classification and the invasiveness of thymic epithelial tumors.[3,4,6,15,27-29] Okumura and colleagues[30] reported that the incidence of invasive tumors associated with Masaoka stages II, III, and IV disease were 13% for type A, 39% for type AB, 40% for type B1, 70% for type B2,

Table 1
WHO histologic classification system

Subtype	Risk	Summary
Type A	Low-risk	Spindle cell; medullary
Type AB		Mixed (type A and type B)
Type B1		Lymphocyte-rich; lymphocytic; predominantly cortical; organoid
Type B2	High-risk	Cortical
Type B3		Epithelial; atypical; squamoid; well-differentiated thymic carcinoma
Thymic carcinoma		Nonorganotypic malignant epithelial neoplasms; lack immature T lymphocyte

Table 2
Masaoka staging system

Stage	Invasion	Description	Survival (%)	
			5-year[a]	20-year[b]
I	Noninvasive	Macroscopically completely encapsulated and microscopically no capsular invasion	96	89
II	Invasive	Microscopic or macroscopic invasion of the surrounding fatty tissue or the mediastinal pleura	86	91
III		Macroscopic invasion of neighboring organs, such as the pericardium, lung, or the great vessels	69	49
IVa		Pericardial or pleural dissemination	50	0
IVb		Lymph node or distant metastases		

[a] 5-year survival.[17]
[b] 20-year survival.[3]

and 80% for type B3 thymomas. According to the multivariate analysis performed by Okumura and colleagues[3] the Masaoka staging system and the WHO histologic classification were independent prognostic factors, whereas the variables of sex, age, association with myasthenia gravis, completeness of resection, and involvement of the great vessels were not prognostic factors. Thus, the WHO histologic classification plays an important role as a prognostic factor, which might result in a helpful tool for making a decision on the treatment strategy.

RADIOGRAPHIC APPEARANCE OF THYMOMAS ACCORDING TO THE WHO HISTOLOGIC CLASSIFICATION

Radiographic imaging such as CT, MRI, and positron emission tomography (PET) is essential for determining treatment strategy for patients with a thymoma. CT, MRI, and PET findings of thymic epithelial tumors classified according to the WHO histologic classification have been mentioned in previous reports.[7–9,31–33] Imaging assessment of thymic epithelial tumors plays an important role in the evaluation and treatment of these patients. However, it is understood that the findings are interpreted as being of limited value in differentiating the various histologic subtypes of thymomas.

CT Findings

According to Tomiyama and colleagues[8] there were no significant differences in size (long- and short-axis diameters) among types A, AB, B1, B2, and B3. In 2 groups based on the long-axis diameters of thymomas (>60 mm and ≤60 mm), there was no significant difference in 5-year survival rates between the low-risk group (types

A, AB, and B1) and high-risk group (types B2 and B3).[31] Regarding the configurations of thymomas on CT, type A thymomas tended to have smooth contours, and the prevalence decreased according to the histologic classification in the order of types A, AB, B1, B2, and B3 (**Figs. 1–5**). There were smaller numbers of tumors with irregular contours in types A, AB, B1, B2, and B3 compared with thymic carcinomas.[8,32] It has been reported that irregular tumor margin is suggestive of capsular invasion of thymoma (ie, invasive thymoma and thymic carcinoma).[34,35]

In terms of the internal nature of thymomas, Sone and colleagues[36] found a higher prevalence of calcification in invasive thymomas. Tomiyama and colleagues[37] reported that calcification was found in 14.5 of 27 cases (54%) of invasive thymomas and 6 of 23 cases (26%) of noninvasive thymomas, and reported that calcification tended to be seen often in types B1, B2, and B3[8] (see **Fig. 4; Fig. 5**A, B). Areas of low attenuation were found significantly more often in patients with invasive thymomas than in patients with noninvasive thymomas.[37] Tumors with a greater malignant potential tend to have areas of low attenuation on CT (see **Fig. 5**C, D). After intravenous administration of contrast material, invasive thymomas showed more heterogeneous attenuation than noninvasive thymomas (see **Fig. 5**).[7,37] Tomiyama and colleagues[37] reported that homogeneous enhancement was found in 11 of 27 cases (41%) of invasive thymoma and 15 of 23 cases (65%) of noninvasive thymoma. Homogeneous enhancement tended to indicate types A or B.[7] Heterogeneous enhancement was more often seen in patients with type B3 thymoma and in those with thymic carcinoma.[7,8] With regard to degree of enhancement, 88% of type A, 86% of type AB,

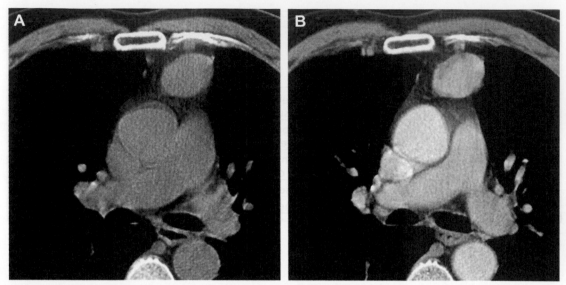

Fig. 1. Type A thymoma unenhanced (*A*) transaxial CT image shows homogeneous anterior mediastinum mass with smooth contours and oval shape. Enhanced (*B*) transaxial CT image shows relatively homogeneous enhanced mass with no contact of adjacent structures. Mass was confirmed histopathologically as type A thymoma (stage I, noninvasive thymoma).

75% of type B3, and 69% of thymic carcinoma showed a high degree of enhancement, and it was more often seen in these tumors (types A, AB, B3, and thymic carcinoma) than in types B1 and B2. One reason for the low enhancement of types B1 and B2 might be that these subtypes of thymoma are both lymphocyte-rich tumors.[8]

Do and colleagues[38] reported that mediastinal lymphadenopathy was found in 4 of 10 cases (40%) of thymic carcinoma and 1 of 12 cases (8%) of invasive thymoma, and thymic carcinoma was more commonly associated with mediastinal nodes than invasive thymoma. Jung and colleagues[39] also reported that lymph node enlargement was significantly found in thymic carcinoma. Mediastinal lymphadenopathy may indicate the greater possibility of thymic carcinoma than any other types of thymoma. Thymic

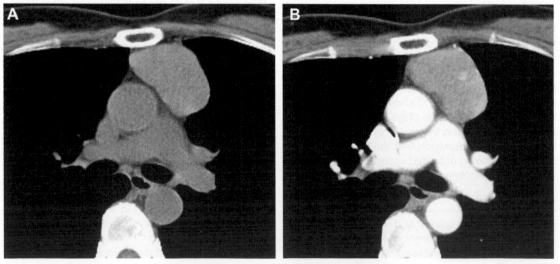

Fig. 2. Type AB thymoma unenhanced (*A*) transaxial CT image shows homogeneous anterior mediastinum mass with slight lobulated margin. Enhanced (*B*) transaxial CT image shows almost homogeneous enhanced mass with no obliteration of fat planes. Mass was confirmed histopathologically as type AB thymoma (stage I, noninvasive thymoma).

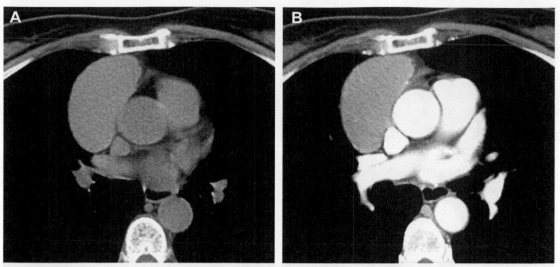

Fig. 3. Type B1 thymoma unenhanced (*A*) transaxial CT image shows homogeneous anterior mediastinum mass with smooth contour. Enhanced (*B*) transaxial CT image shows almost homogeneous enhanced mass in contact with the right side of ascending aorta and superior vena cava. Note no obliteration of fat planes. Mass was confirmed histopathologically as type B1 thymoma (stage I, noninvasive thymoma).

carcinomas have a greater tendency to invade the great vessels, to develop distant metastases, and to cause phrenic nerve palsy than any other types of thymoma.[7,8] Pleural dissemination is seen in type B and thymic carcinoma (see **Fig. 5**C, D), but not in types A or AB.[38,39] Although invasion of adjacent structures was suggested when the tumor widely abutted the adjacent tissue or when

an area with a fat density between tumor and adjacent tissue visually disappeared on CT, partial or complete obliteration of fat planes around the tumor was not helpful in distinguishing invasive from noninvasive thymomas.[37] Tomiyama and colleagues[37] reported that infiltration of adjacent mediastinal structures was suggested on CT in all patients with surgically proved mediastinal

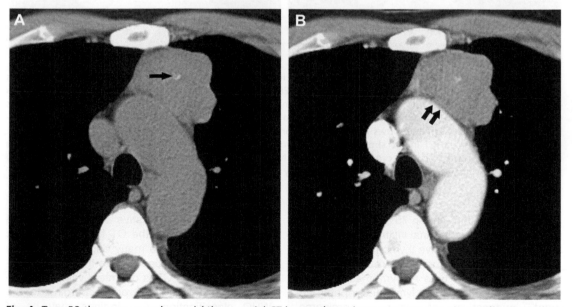

Fig. 4. Type B2 thymoma unenhanced (*A*) transaxial CT image shows homogeneous anterior mediastinum mass with lobulated margin and tiny calcification (*arrow*). Enhanced (*B*) transaxial CT image shows homogeneous enhanced mass in contact with aortic arch. Note partial obliteration of fat planes (*arrows*). Mass was confirmed histopathologically as type B2 thymoma (stage III, invasive thymoma).

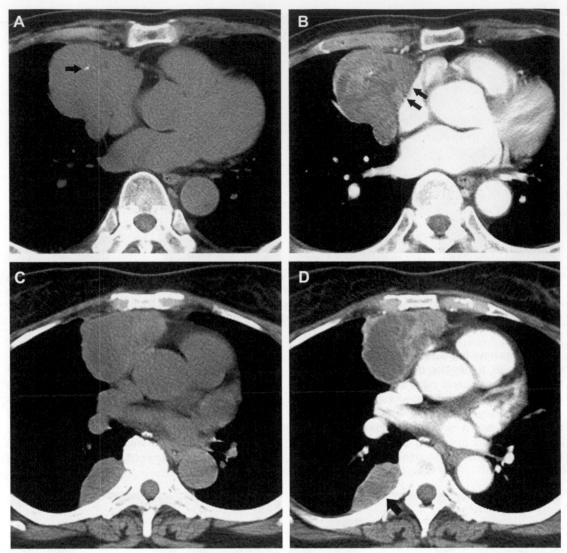

Fig. 5. Type B3 thymoma unenhanced (*A*) transaxial CT image shows heterogeneous anterior mediastinum mass with lobulated margin and tiny calcification (*arrow*). Enhanced (*B*) transaxial CT image shows heterogeneous enhanced mass in contact with right atrium. Note almost complete obliteration of fat planes (*arrows*). Mass was confirmed histopathologically as type B3 thymoma (stage III, invasive thymoma). Type B3 thymoma unenhanced (*C*) transaxial CT image shows heterogeneous anterior mediastinum mass with slight lobulated margin. Enhanced (*D*) transaxial CT image shows heterogeneous enhanced mass with low attenuation area, which is considered to be a necrosis or a cystic degeneration. Note pleural dissemination in right paravertebral (Th7) region (*arrow*). Mass was confirmed histopathologically as type B3 thymoma (stage IV, invasive thymoma).

structural infiltration, and in 75% of invasive thymomas with no mediastinal infiltration at surgery and in 40% of noninvasive thymomas.

Thus, smooth contours and a round shape are most suggestive of type A thymomas. Irregular contours and mediastinal lymphadenopathy are most suggestive of thymic carcinoma. Calcification is suggestive of type B1, B2, and B3 thymomas. The combination of homogeneous enhancement and a high degree of enhancement is suggestive of type A and AB thymomas. However, the CT findings of thymic epithelial tumors have many degrees of overlap among subgroups according to the WHO classification. Although CT is of limited value in differentiating histologic subtypes according to the WHO classification, CT findings may be of some use for predicting postoperative recurrence or metastasis in patients with thymic epithelial tumors.

MR Findings

There are few reports of the MR findings of thymic epithelial tumors based on the WHO classification.[7,32,33,40–44] Type A, AB, and B1 thymomas (low-risk group) showed signal intensity similar to or slightly higher than that of muscle on T1-weighted images, and showed signal intensity higher than that of muscle but similar to that of fatty tissue on T2-weighted images (**Fig. 6**).[40–44] Type A, AB, and B1 thymomas tended to show homogeneous and moderate enhancement on gadopentetate dimeglumine-enhanced (Gd) T1-weighted images. The signal intensity of type B2 and B3 thymomas is almost the same as that of type A, AB, and B1 thymomas on both T1- and T2-weighted image.[43,44] However, T2-weighted images of most type B2 and B3 thymomas often show heterogeneous signal intensities with scattered high-intensity areas. These findings are believed to correspond to cystic spaces with or without hemorrhage.[7,43] Moreover, in cases with calcifications, T2-weighted images often show low signal intensity in tumors. Except for calcification, low signal intensity on T2-weighted imaging usually indicates lesions with flow voids (fluids with rapid or turbulent flow), hemorrhage (deoxyhemoglobin or hemosiderin), or fibrosis.[45,46] Although some type B2 and B3 thymomas have histologic architectural features such as perivascular spaces and perivascular arrangement of tumor cells,[1] it may be difficult to detect these microstructures on MR images. However, Sakai and colleagues[43] reported that 11 of 12 malignant thymomas were visualized as having heterogeneous signal intensity on T2-weighted images, corresponding to the presence of cystic or hemorrhagic regions noted pathologically. Visualization of a heterogeneous intensity on T2-weighted images suggests a high-risk thymoma (**Fig. 7**). On the other hand, thymic carcinomas show low signal intensity on both T1- and T2-weighted MR images; in particular, there is a higher prevalence of low-signal foci within the mass on T2-weighted images than for any other types of thymoma.[33,44] Kushihashi and colleagues[44] reported that thymic carcinomas contained abundant collagenous tissue, which may result in the low signal intensity on T2-weighted images.

In the pathologic specimens, fibrous septa can sometimes be found in type AB, B1, B2, and B3 thymomas.[1,33] Fibrous septa can be detected as low-signal bands (septa) on T2-weighted images.[7,43] Although it is difficult to distinguish the histologic subtypes from the presence of septa, Sakai and colleagues[43] reported that the presence of sharply defined fibrous septa dividing tumors into lobules is one of the most characteristic features of thymomas. In addition, the finding of an almost complete capsule was seen on MR images of thymomas (see **Fig. 6**) but not of thymic carcinomas. Sadohara and colleagues[32] reported that the presence of a capsule and septum on MRI is useful for differentiating thymic carcinomas

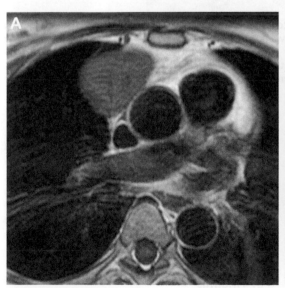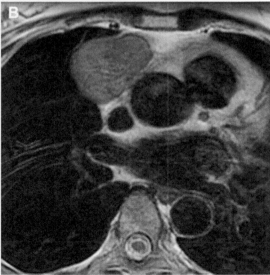

Fig. 6. Typical MR image of noninvasive thymoma T1-weighted image (*A*) shows signal intensity similar to or slightly higher than that of muscle, whereas T2-weighted image (*B*) shows signal intensity higher than that of muscle. Note low-signal rim as the presence of a capsule on T2-weighted image (*B*) and no invasion of adjacent structures. Mass was confirmed histopathologically as type B1 thymoma (stage I, noninvasive thymoma).

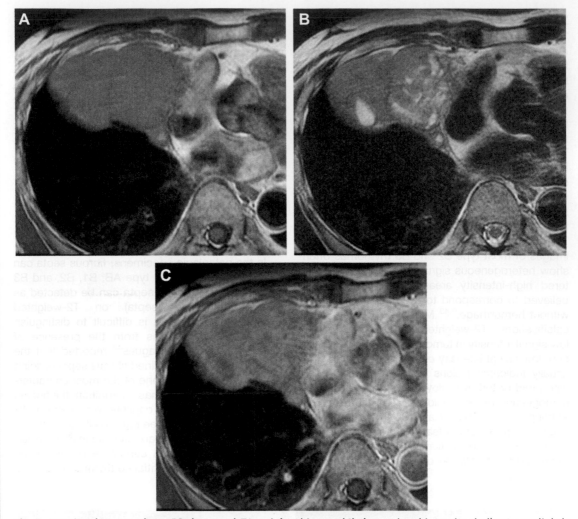

Fig. 7. Invasive thymoma (type B3 thymoma) T1-weighted image (*A*) shows signal intensity similar to or slightly higher than that of muscle. T2-weighted image (*B*) shows heterogeneous signal intensity mass with intratumor high-signal areas, which are considered to be cystic components because of no enhancement on Gd-T1-weighted image (*C*). Note that MR images (*A, B, C*) are strongly suggestive of tumor invasion to the pericardium. Mass was confirmed histopathologically as type B3 thymoma (stage III, invasive thymoma).

from thymomas. Furthermore, the absence of a capsule on MRI is strongly suggestive of tumor invasion to the surrounding tissue. With regard to tumor invasion of a great vessel, which is a significant predictor for poor prognosis,[47] the presence of great-vessel invasion is an important feature in diagnosing thymic carcinoma because thymic carcinomas have a higher prevalence of great-vessel invasion than thymomas.[9,32]

On MR images, the tumors with smooth contours, an almost complete capsule, the presence of a septum, and homogeneous enhancement are more likely to be low-risk thymomas than high-risk thymomas or thymic carcinomas. MRI findings such as heterogeneous and

intratumor low-signal foci on T2-weighted images, heterogeneous signal intensity on T1-weighted images, pleural effusion, and lymphadenopathy may be suggestive of a high-risk thymoma. Although MRI may be more useful for evaluating the internal structure of tumor and the presence of tumor invasion than CT, MRI is also of limited value in differentiating among histologic subtypes according to the WHO classification.

PET Findings

It has been reported that [^{18}F]fluorodeoxyglucose (FDG)-PET scan might prove to be useful for differentiating thymic carcinoma from other entities within the thymus.[48,49] Sung and colleagues[50] reported that the maximum standard uptake value (SUV$_{max}$) of thymomas (median 5.5 in high-risk thymomas [types B2 and B3] and median 3.9 in low-risk thymomas [types A, AB, and B1]) was significantly lower than that of thymic carcinoma (median 9.1). However, the usefulness of FDG-PET may be equivocal in regard to differentiation between invasive and noninvasive thymomas and also between thymomas and thymic hyperplasia.[51] Many reports have shown that delayed imaging with dual-phase FDG-PET was advantageous for diagnosing malignant tumors.[52] Demura and colleagues[52] suggested that dual-phase FDG-PET imaging was useful for differentiating malignant thorax lesions from benign lesions. A recent report assessed the usefulness of dual-phase FDG-PET for the diagnosis of the various subtypes of thymic epithelial tumors based on the WHO classification.[53] Inoue and colleagues[53] reported that the early SUV$_{max}$ cutoff value of 6.2 appeared to be useful for differentiating between thymomas

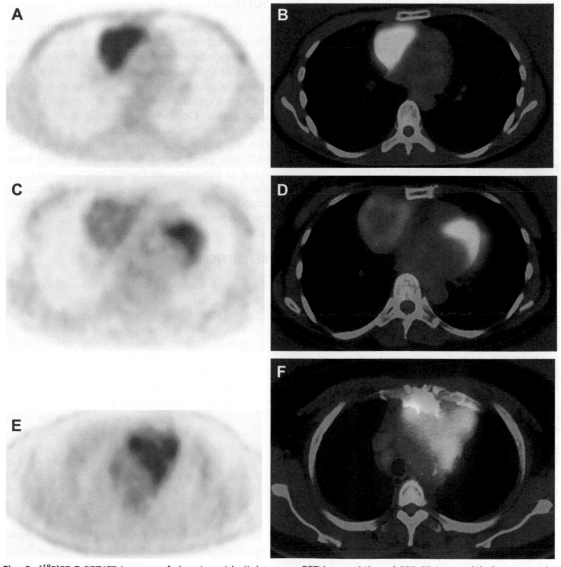

Fig. 8. [^{18}F]FDG-PET/CT images of thymic epithelial tumors PET image (*A*) and PET-CT image (*B*) show anterior mediastinum mass with SUV$_{max}$ value of 5.4. Mass was confirmed histopathologically as type AB thymoma. PET image (*C*) and PET-CT image (*D*) show anterior mediastinum mass with SUV$_{max}$ value of 2.6. Mass was confirmed histopathologically as type B1 thymoma. PET image (*E*) and PET-CT image (*F*) show anterior mediastinum mass with SUV$_{max}$ value of 7.8 and right paratracheal lymph node with SUV$_{max}$ value of 2.3 (*arrow*). Mass was confirmed histopathologically as thymic carcinoma.

and thymic carcinoma (sensitivity, 63.6%; specificity, 91.4%; and accuracy, 84.8%), and that early SUV_{max} values greater than 7.1 could completely differentiate thymic carcinomas from thymomas (types A, AB, B1, B2, and B3) (**Fig. 8**). The delayed SUV values tended to be higher than the early SUV values in all types of thymic epithelial tumors, indicating no significant advantages for differentiating tumors. Moreover, Inoue and colleagues reported that the early SUV_{max} cutoff value of 4.5 might differentiate between low-risk thymomas (types A, AB, and B1) and high-risk thymomas (types B2, B3, and thymic carcinoma) based on the WHO classification. This information may be useful to predict the prognosis of thymic epithelial tumors, despite some limitations in clearly distinguishing between the various subtypes of tumors. On the other hand, some reports showed that there was no difference in FDG uptake between invasive thymomas and noninvasive thymomas.[51] Therefore, general examination by multimodality (CT, MRI, and PET) is believed to be important before recommending pretreatment biopsy, such as a CT-guided percutaneous cutting needle biopsy (PCNB) or surgery/open biopsy.

HISTOLOGIC EXAMINATION AND DIAGNOSIS OF THYMIC EPITHELIAL TUMORS

CT is commonly used in biopsies to assist with precision guidance of the instruments necessary to perform the biopsy to the appropriate area of the body. CT-guided PCNB is often preferred because most mediastinal tumors are located adjacent to major blood vessels and other important structures.[54] In addition, Yanagawa and colleagues[55] reported that CT-guided PCNB was a technique with a good concordance of the WHO classification of thymic epithelial tumors between the diagnoses of surgery/open biopsy. The diagnosis by CT and/or MRI was prone to an overdiagnosis or an underdiagnosis. Even when the simplified WHO classification, which was grouped into 4 categories (types A and AB, type B1, types B2 and B3, and thymic carcinoma), was used, the concordance between the diagnosis of CT and that of surgical resection specimens classified according to the simplified WHO classification was only moderate.[55] Conversely, some reports showed high concordance between the diagnosis established by CT-guided PCNB and the diagnosis of the surgical specimen in patients with a thymic epithelial tumor classified according to the WHO classification.[55,56] Thus, CT-guided PCNB is a reliable procedure for the diagnosis of thymic epithelial tumors in accordance with the WHO classification, and in

particular might be more useful for histopathologic diagnosis in patients with nonresectable tumors. Herman and colleagues[57] have reported difficulty in differentiating thymomas from malignant lymphomas. Considering that immunohistochemical examination enables the diagnosis of mediastinal lymphoma[58] and the differentiation between thymic carcinomas and thymomas,[59] the combination of CT-guided PCNB of thymic epithelial tumors and immunohistochemical analysis provides more accurate diagnoses.

SUMMARY

This article presents the radiographic criteria and the characteristics of thymomas and reviews the clinical significance of the WHO histologic classification of thymic epithelial tumors. The histologic appearance of thymic epithelial tumors reflects the oncologic behavior of thymomas and thymic carcinomas. Comprehension of imaging findings of thymic epithelial tumors according to the WHO histologic classification on CT, MRI, and FDG-PET may provide helpful assessment and treatment of patients with thymic epithelial tumors in the clinical setting. However, diagnosis from only imaging findings is of limited value in differentiating the various histologic subtypes of thymomas.

REFERENCES

1. Rosai J, Sobin LH. Histological typing of tumours of the thymus. International histological classification of tumours. 2nd edition. New York: Springer; 1999.
2. Travis WD, Brambilla E, Muller-Hermelink HK, et al. Editors, Pathology and genetics: tumors of the lung, pleura, thymus and heart. Lyon (France): IARC; 2004.
3. Okumura M, Ohta M, Tateyama H, et al. The World Health Organization histologic classification system reflects the oncological behavior of thymoma: a clinical study of 273 patients. Cancer 2002;94(3): 624–32.
4. Chen G, Marx A, Wen-Hu C, et al. New WHO histologic classification predicts prognosis of thymic epithelial tumors: a clinicopathologic study of 200 thymoma cases from China. Cancer 2002;95(2): 420–9.
5. Chalabreysse L, Roy P, Cordier JF, et al. Correlation of the WHO schema for the classification of thymic epithelial neoplasms with prognosis: a retrospective study of 90 tumors. Am J Surg Pathol 2002;26(12): 1605–11.
6. Kondo K, Yoshizawa K, Tsuyuguchi M, et al. WHO histologic classification is a prognostic indicator in thymoma. Ann Thorac Surg 2004;77(4):1183–8.

7. Han J, Lee KS, Yi CA, et al. Thymic epithelial tumors classified according to a newly established WHO scheme: CT and MR findings. Korean J Radiol 2003;4(8):46–53.

8. Tomiyama N, Johkoh T, Mihara N, et al. Using The World Health Organization classification of thymic epithelial neoplasms to describe CT findings. AJR Am J Roentgenol 2002;179(24):881–6.

9. Jeong YJ, Lee KS, Kim J, et al. Does CT of thymic epithelial tumors enable us to differentiate histologic subtypes and predict prognosis? AJR Am J Roentgenol 2004;183(14):283–9.

10. Suster S, Moran CA. Micronodular thymoma with lymphoid B-cell hyperplasia: clinicopathologic and immunohistochemical study of eighteen cases of a distinctive morphologic variant of thymic epithelial neoplasm. Am J Surg Pathol 1999;23:955–62.

11. Tateyama H, Saito Y, Fujii Y, et al. The spectrum of micronodular thymic epithelial tumours with lymphoid B-cell hyperplasia. Histopathology 2001; 38:519–27.

12. Suster S, Moran CA, Chan JK. Thymoma with pseudosarcomatous stroma: report of an unusual histologic variant of thymic epithelial neoplasm that may simulate carcinosarcoma. Am J Surg Pathol 1997; 21:1316–23.

13. Yoneda S, Marx A, Heimann S, et al. Low-grade metaplastic carcinoma of the thymus. Histopathology 1999;35:19–30.

14. Kuo T. Sclerosing thymoma—a possible phenomenon of regression. Histopathology 1994;25: 289–91.

15. Okumura M, Miyoshi S, Fujii Y, et al. Clinical and functional significance of WHO classification of human thymic epithelial neoplasms. A study of 146 consecutive tumors. Am J Surg Pathol 2001;25: 103–10.

16. Giaccone G, Wilmink H, Paul MA, et al. Systemic treatment of malignant thymoma. Am J Clin Oncol 2006;29(4):336–44.

17. Masaoka A, Monden Y, Nakahara K, et al. Follow-up study of thymomas with special reference to their clinical stages. Cancer 1981;48:2485–92.

18. Nakahara K, Ohno K, Hashimoto J, et al. Thymoma: results with complete resection and adjuvant postoperative irradiation in 141 consecutive patients. J Thorac Cardiovasc Surg 1988;95:1041–7.

19. Regnard JF, Magdeleinat P, Dromer C, et al. Prognostic factors and long-term results after thymoma resection: a series of 307 patients. J Thorac Cardiovasc Surg 1996;112:376–84.

20. Maggi G, Casadio C, Cavallo A, et al. Thymoma: results of 241 operated cases. Ann Thorac Surg 1991;51:152–6.

21. Wilkins KB, Sheikh E, Green R, et al. Clinical and pathologic predictors of survival in patients with thymoma. Ann Surg 1999;230:562–74.

22. Wilkins EW Jr, Edmunds LH, Castleman B. Cases of thymoma at the Massachusetts General Hospital. J Thorac Cardiovasc Surg 1966;52:322–30.

23. Monden Y, Nakahara K, Kagotani K, et al. Myasthenia gravis with thymoma: analysis of and postoperative prognosis for 65 patients with thymomatous myasthenia gravis. Ann Thorac Surg 1984;38: 46–52.

24. Wilkins EW Jr, Grillo HC, Scannell JG, et al. Role of staging in prognosis and management of thymoma. Ann Thorac Surg 1991;51:888–92.

25. Blumberg D, Port JL, Weksler B, et al. Thymoma: a multivariate analysis of factors predicting survival. Ann Thorac Surg 1995;60:908–14.

26. Okumura M, Miyoshi S, Takeuchi Y, et al. Results of surgical treatment of thymomas with special reference to the involved organs. J Thorac Cardiovasc Surg 1999;117:605–13.

27. Nakagawa K, Asamura H, Matsuno Y, et al. Thymoma: a clinicopathologic study based on the new World Health Organization classification. J Thorac Cardiovasc Surg 2003;126:1134–40.

28. Park MS, Chung KY, Kim KD, et al. Prognosis of thymic epithelial tumors according to the new World Health Organization histologic classification. Ann Thorac Surg 2004;78:992–7.

29. Kim DJ, Yang WI, Choi SS, et al. Prognostic and clinical relevance of the World Health Organization schema for the classification of thymic epithelial tumors: a clinicopathologic study of 108 patients and literature review. Chest 2005;127:755–61.

30. Okumura M, Shiono H, Minami M, et al. Clinical and pathological aspects of thymic epithelial tumors. Gen Thorac Cardiovasc Surg 2008;56:10–6.

31. Yakushiji S, Tateishi U, Nagai S, et al. Computed tomographic findings and prognosis in thymic epithelial tumor patients. J Comput Assist Tomogr 2008;32(5):799–805.

32. Sadohara J, Fujimoto K, Müller NL, et al. Thymic epithelial tumors: comparison of CT and MR imaging findings of low-risk thymomas, high-risk thymomas, and thymic carcinomas. Eur J Radiol 2006;60:70–9.

33. Inoue A, Tomiyama N, Fujimoto K, et al. MR imaging of thymic epithelial tumors: correlation with World Health Organization classification. Radiat Med 2006;24:171–81.

34. Rosado-de-Christenson ML, Galobardes J, Moran CA. Thymoma: radiologic–pathologic correlation. Radiographics 1992;12:151–68.

35. Strollo DC, Rosado-de-Christenson ML. Tumors of the thymus. J Thorac Imaging 1999;14:152–71.

36. Sone S, Higashihara T, Morimoto S, et al. [CT of thymoma]. Nippon Igaku Hoshasen Gakkai Zasshi 1982;42:731–9 [in Japanese].

37. Tomiyama N, Müller NL, Ellis SJ, et al. Invasive and non-invasive thymoma: distinctive CT features. J Comput Assist Tomogr 2001;25:388–93.

38. Do YS, Im JG, Lee BH, et al. CT findings in malignant tumors of thymic epithelium. J Comput Assist Tomogr 1995;19:192–7.

39. Jung KJ, Lee KS, Han J, et al. Malignant thymic epithelial tumors: CT–pathologic correlation. AJR Am J Roentgenol 2001;176:433–9.

40. Herold CJ, Zerhouni EA. The mediastinum and lungs. In: Higgins CB, Hricak H, Helms CA, editors. Magnetic resonance imaging of the body. 2nd edition. NewYork: Raven Press; 1992.

41. Molina PL, Siegel MJ, Glazer HS. Thymic masses on MR imaging. AJR Am J Roentgenol 1990;155:495–500.

42. Ikezoe J, Takeuchi N, Johkoh T, et al. MRI of anterior mediastinal tumors. Radiat Med 1992;10:176–83.

43. Sakai F, Sone S, Kiyono K, et al. MR imaging of thymoma: radiologic-pathologic correlation. AJR Am J Roentgenol 1992;158:751–6.

44. Kushihashi T, Fujisawa H, Munechika H. Magnetic resonance imaging of thymic epithelial tumors. Crit Rev Diagn Imaging 1996;37:191–259.

45. Warakaulle DR, Anslow P. Differential diagnosis of intracranial lesions with high signal on T1 or low signal on T2-weighted MRI. Clin Radiol 2003;58: 922–33.

46. Yamato M, Nishimura G, Koguchi Y, et al. Calcified leiomyoma of deep soft tissue in a child. Pediatr Radiol 1999;29:135–7.

47. Tseng YL, Wang ST, Wu MH, et al. Thymic carcinoma: involvement of great vessels indicates poor prognosis. Ann Thorac Surg 2003;76:1041–6.

48. Ferdinand B, Gupta P, Kramer EL. Spectrum of thymic uptake at 18F-FDG PET. Radiographics 2004;24:1611–6.

49. Patel PM, Alibazoglu H, Ali A, et al. Normal thymic uptake of FDG on PET imaging. Clin Nucl Med 1996;21:772–5.

50. Sung YM, Lee KS, Kim BT, et al. 18FFDG PET/CT of thymic epithelial tumors: usefulness for distinguishing and staging tumor subgroups. J Nucl Med 2006;47:1628–34.

51. Sasaki M, Kuwabara Y, Ichiya Y, et al. Differential diagnosis of thymic tumors using a combination of 11C-methionine PET and FDG PET. J Nucl Med 1999;40:1595–601.

52. Demura Y, Tsuchida T, Ishizaki T, et al. 18F-FDG accumulation with PET for differentiation between benign and malignant lesions in the thorax. J Nucl Med 2003;44:540–8.

53. Inoue A, Tomiyama N, Tatsumi M, et al. 18F-FDG PET for the evaluation of thymic epithelial tumors: correlation with the World Health Organization classification in addition to dual-time-point imaging. Eur J Nucl Med Mol Imaging 2009;36:1219–25.

54. Klein JS, Salomon G, Stewart EA. Transthoracic needle biopsy with a coaxially placed 20-gauge automated cutting needle: results in 122 patients. Radiology 1996;198(3):715–20.

55. Yanagawa M, Tomiyama N, Honda O, et al. CT-guided percutaneous cutting needle biopsy of thymic epithelial tumors: comparison to the accuracy of computed tomographic diagnosis according to the World Health Organization classification. Acad Radiol 2010;17(6):772–8.

56. Yonemori K, Tsuta K, Tateishi U, et al. Diagnostic accuracy of CT-guided percutaneous cutting needle biopsy for thymic tumours. Clin Radiol 2006;61(9): 771–5.

57. Herman SJ, Holub RV, Weisbrod GL, et al. Anterior mediastinal masses: utility of transthoracic needle biopsy. Radiology 1991;180(1):167–70.

58. Suster S. Primary large-cell lymphomas of the mediastinum. Semin Diagn Pathol 1999;16(1):51–64.

59. Pan CC, Chen PC, Chiang H. KIT (CD117) is frequently overexpressed in thymic carcinomas but is absent in thymomas. J Pathol 2004;202(3): 375–81.

Neuroendocrine Tumors of the Thymus

Enrico Ruffini, MD[a],*, Alberto Oliaro, MD[b],
Domenico Novero, MD[c], Paola Campisi, MD[c],
Pier Luigi Filosso, MD[a]

KEYWORDS

- Thymus • Mediastinum • Neuroendocrine tumors
- Surgery • Pathology

Primary neuroendocrine tumors of the thymus (NETTs) are rare neoplasms that were misdiagnosed as thymomas until 1972, when Rosai and Higa[1] first described the existence of carcinoid tumors in the thymic gland, thus separating these neoplasms from thymomas. Since then, about 250 cases of primary NETTs have been described in the literature: most are case reports, and only a few small clinical series have been reported.[2–15] Most of these single-center studies are too small to provide a uniform assessment of the various treatment modalities and of the factors influencing survival.

This article is an updated review of incidence, clinical presentation, histology, treatment options, and survival of patients with primary NETT.

INCIDENCE, CLINICAL PRESENTATION, AND DIAGNOSIS

NETTs are rare neoplasms with an overall age-adjusted incidence of 0.01/100.000 per year.[4] It has been estimated that NETTs account for 2% to 4% of all anterior mediastinal tumors.[2,3] Virtually all primary mediastinal NE tumors arise in the thymus[16]; primary NETTs must be differentiated from other mediastinal thymic tumors (**Box 1**).[17] Primary NETTs are predominantly located in the anterior mediastinum, although exceptional cases have been described in the middle or posterior compartments; sometimes, because of the tumor extent, the neoplasm can occupy all 3 compartments.[18,19] Previous series used the term carcinoid to indicate these tumors; however, NETTs, contrary to well-differentiated carcinoid tumors, frequently present atypical histologic features,[9] and they should therefore be considered as belonging to the spectrum of NE carcinomas; most investigators[3,11,13,14] correlated patients' survival with tumor differentiation. It is therefore recommended not to use the term carcinoid for these neoplasms.

NETTs show a predominance for men, with a male/female ratio of about 3:1[20]; the mean age at presentation is 54 years, ranging from 16 to 97 years.

Tumors are asymptomatic in only 30% of cases,[17] usually discovered incidentally after routine chest radiograph. More frequently, patients present with nonspecific symptoms (cough, chest pain, shortness of breath, weight loss, asthenia, chronic fever) or superior vena cava syndrome.

Chest radiograph is usually not specific; computed tomography and magnetic resonance imaging (MRI) offer a detailed imaging of the tumor and its extent to the surrounding structures.[21] Computed tomography and MRI findings in NETTs include large, lobulated, and generally locally invasive anterior mediastinal masses with areas of focal hemorrhage and/or necrosis (**Fig. 1**).[5,17] The presence of somatostatin receptors within the neoplastic tissue justifies the use of [111]indium-diethylenetriamine pentaacetic acid-D-phenylalanine-octreotide (Octreoscan) scintigraphy not only for preoperative assessment but

a Division of Thoracic Surgery, University of Torino, Via Genova, 3, 10126 Torino, Italy
b Head of the Division of Thoracic Surgery, University of Torino, Via Genova, 3, 10126 Torino, Italy
c Division of Pathology, University of Torino, Corso Bramante, 88–90, 10126 Torino, Italy
* Corresponding author.
E-mail address: enrico.ruffini@unito.it

Thorac Surg Clin 21 (2011) 13–23
doi:10.1016/j.thorsurg.2010.08.013
1547-4127/11/$ — see front matter © 2011 Elsevier Inc. All rights reserved.

also during follow-up.[14,22] Octreotide selectively binds to subtype 2 somatostatin receptors (sst$_2$), which are the most frequently expressed receptors in NE tumors, especially in typical carcinoids.[23,24] Positron emission tomography (PET) scan and integrated PET-computed tomography have been found to be useful in the diagnosis and preoperative staging of NETTs[25]; Cardillo and colleagues[14] recommend PET scan for preoperative workup, along with computed tomography, MRI, and Octreoscan.

Thymic NE tumors show a more aggressive biologic behavior than their lung or abdominal counterparts, and an advanced stage at presentation is more frequent in NETTs than in other NE tumors. Duh and colleagues[26] reported that NETTs are malignant in about 80% of cases compared with 25% in bronchial carcinoids. Valli and colleagues[7] and de Montpreville and colleagues[9] suggested that NETTs behave similarly to the atypical carcinoid form of NE tumors of the lung according to Arrigoni and colleagues'[27] classification. de Montpreville and colleagues[9] found that typical carcinoids are exceptional in the thymus and most NETTs are moderately or poorly differentiated NE carcinomas, corresponding to the atypical carcinoids or the small-cell carcinomas of the previous classification. As a consequence, up to 30% of patients with NETTs have metastases at presentation, mostly to the liver, brain, bones, head, and neck.[28,29]

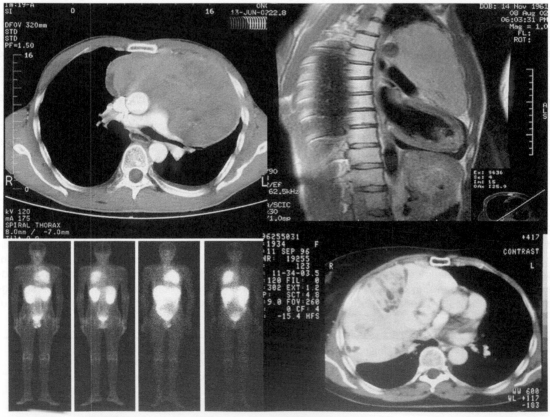

Fig. 1. Radiologic imaging (chest computed tomography, MRI, and Octreoscan) in a patient with NETT.

As observed in most NE malignancies, NETTs are associated with endocrinopathies, of which the most frequent are: Cushing syndrome (30% of cases) and multiple endocrine neoplasia type 1 (MEN-1) syndrome (10%–25% of cases); rarely, prolactin secretion, hyperparathyroidism, von Recklinghausen, and MEN-2 syndrome (incomplete Sipple syndrome) have been described.[12,14,30] When associated with Cushing syndrome, NETTs occur as frequently in men as in women, with an age peak between the second and the fourth decades of life[12]; in these patients tumors are usually larger, more locally invasive, and more aggressive than in NETTs without Cushing syndrome. In patients with MEN-1, NETTs are less common than parathyroid or enteropancreatic and anterior pituitary tumors.[28] Less common paraneoplastic conditions and systemic manifestations associated with NETTs include polyarthropathy, peripheral neuropathy, proximal myopathy, hypertrophic osteoarthropathy, and Eaton Lambert syndrome.[31,32] The association between NETTs and myasthenia gravis is rare, with only one case reported in the English literature.[33] Unlike carcinoid tumors of the lung and the gastrointestinal tract, carcinoid syndrome is exceptional and only 2 cases have been described so far.[34]

HISTOLOGY
Histologic Classification

According to the World Health Organization (WHO) NETTs are defined as "epithelial tumors predominantly or exclusively composed of neuroendocrine cells," taking into account that otherwise typical thymic carcinoma may contain scattered NE cells.

Different histologic classifications of NE tumors are in use because a definitive correlation between morphologic aspects and biologic behavior has not been found so far. The 2 most used classifications are the WHO and the Armed Forces Institute of Pathology (AFIP).

The WHO classification[35] categorizes NE tumors in **Table 1**:

1) Well-differentiated NE carcinomas including typical and atypical carcinoids. The former include tumor cells with minimal cytologic atypias, disposed in organoid pattern (nests, ribbons, or festoons) with fewer than 2 mitoses per 10 high-power field (HPF) and absent necrosis. Conversely, atypical carcinoids show the same morphologic features of typical carcinoid, but with a greater mitotic index (between 2 and 10 mitoses per 10 HPF) and/or necrosis.

2) Poorly differentiated NE carcinomas including small-cell carcinoma and large-cell carcinoma. Small-cell carcinoma is composed of cells with scant cytoplasm, granular chromatin, inconspicuous nucleoli, and a high mitotic rate (>10 mitoses per 10 HPF). Large-cell carcinoma includes tumors consisting of large cells with cytologic NE features, arranged in nests or trabeculae. Diffuse and abundant necrosis and a high number of mitoses (>10 per 10 HPF) are common.

The AFIP classification proposed by Suster and Moran[36] includes a 3-grade classification of NE tumors into well, moderately, and poorly differentiated forms.[15,37] The correspondence between the WHO and AFIP classifications is shown in **Table 2**.

Unusual histologic variants mostly resembling other solid-organ neoplasms are of less common observation and include[35]:

Oncocytic carcinoid: tumor cells are large and eosinophilic with abundant granular cytoplasms rich in mitochondria

Spindle cell carcinoid: partially or totally composed of spindle cells organized in fascicles

Pigmented carcinoid: characterized by deposition of melanin in intracellular (in a variable number of cells) and extracellular

Table 1
Histologic criteria for NE tumors of the thymus

	Typical Carcinoma	Atypical Carcinoma	Small-cell Carcinoma
Mitoses per 100 HPFs	<10	>10	Any
Necrosis	Absent	Present	Present
Pleomorphism	Minimal	Moderate	Moderate
Nuclear molding	None	Minimal	Prominent
Crush artifact	None	Minimal	Prominent

Data from Gal AA, Kornstein MJ, Cohen C, et al. Neuroendocrine tumors of the thymus: a clinicopathologic and prognostic study. Ann Thorac Surg 2001;72:1179–82.

Table 2
Comparison of WHO and AFIP classification of NETTs

WHO	AFIP
Well-differentiated NE tumors Typical carcinoid	Well-differentiated (low-grade) NE carcinoma
Atypical carcinoid	Moderately differentiated (intermediate-grade) NE carcinoma
Poorly differentiated NE tumors	Poorly differentiated (high-grade) NE carcinoma Small-cell NE carcinoma Large-cell NE carcinoma

Data from Suster S, Moran CA. Neuroendocrine neoplasms of the mediastinum. Am J Clin Pathol 2001;115 Suppl:S17–27; Moran CA. Primary neuroendocrine carcinomas of the mediastinum: review of current criteria for histopathologic diagnosis and classification. Semin Diagn Pathol 2005;22(3):223–9.

(melanophages) location. Metastasis of melanocytic tumors needs to be ruled out

Mucinous carcinoid: a rare variant composed of tumor cells arranged in nests or small clusters among mucinous stroma of sulfated acid mucopolysaccharides (positive with Alcian-blue staining). Differential diagnosis is imperative, with metastasis of mucus-producing tumors

Angiomatoid carcinoid: tumor cells form dilated cystic spaces filled with blood. Vascular tumors need to be ruled out

Carcinoid with amyloidlike stroma[15]: islands of files of tumor cells are embedded in fibrosclerotic connectival stroma. This variant resembles medullary carcinoma of thyroid. Because some carcinoids produce calcitonin, differentiating between the 2 neoplasms can be difficult

Carcinoid with sarcomatous changes: tumor composed of both NE cells and sarcomatous elements, which can be of fibrous, myoid, osseous, or chondroid origin.

Macroscopic aspects

Macroscopically, NETTs are generally not encapsulated tumors with an aggressive behavior toward surrounding organs. Dimensions vary between 2 and 20 cm. On cut section they appear of gray-white color and firm consistency. Foci of necrosis or hemorrhage can be found.

Microscopic Aspects

Well-differentiated tumors are composed of monotonous cells with abundant cytoplasm, small round nuclei, finely distributed nuclear chromatin, and inconspicuous nucleoli. Areas of necrosis (also comedolike necrosis) and dystrophic calcifications are common in atypical carcinoids. Cells are arranged in nests, rosettalike structures, trabeculae, or festoons (**Figs. 2** and **3**). In less

differentiated tumors cells can be disposed in sheets or in file among desmoplastic stroma.

Poorly differentiated NETTs are characterized by large (large-cell carcinoma) or small (small-cell carcinoma) cells with marked cytologic atypias (**Fig. 4**) and nuclear chromatin fragility, which is the cause of common streaking artifact of nuclear material.[38] Often organoid architecture is lost and it is difficult to recognize NE origin in these neoplasms. Extensive areas of necrosis and cellular debris are common. High mitotic rate (>10 mitoses per 10 HPF) is always observed. Small-cell and large-cell carcinoma need to be distinguished from their pulmonary counterparts.

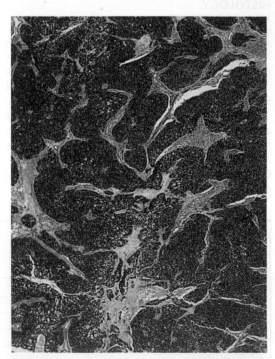

Fig. 2. Atypical carcinoid: cells are arranged in nests and islands (hematoxylin-eosin, original magnification ×2).

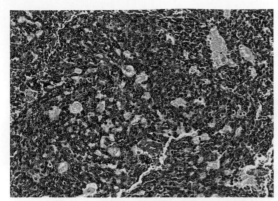

Fig. 3. Atypical carcinoid: cells are arranged in roset-talike pattern (hematoxylin-eosin, original magnification ×10).

As pulmonary neoplasms are more common, it is important to rule out this possibility, before making a diagnosis of primitive NETTs.[36]

Immunohistochemical Findings

Immunohistochemistry is of primary importance to confirm the NE origin of NETTs. NE immunohistochemical markers include chromogranin A (**Fig. 5**), synaptophysin, neuron-specific enolase, and CD56. NETTs are positive for broad-spectrum cytokeratin (AE1/AE3 or CAM 5.2) with a typical dot-like pattern (**Fig. 6**). Expression of hormones is variable: adrenocorticotropic hormone, somatostatin, cholecystokinin, calcitonin, and gastrin can be produced by tumor cells.

TREATMENT AND SURVIVAL

A preoperative histologic diagnosis should be obtained particularly in those patients presenting with symptoms of locally invasive disease, in the

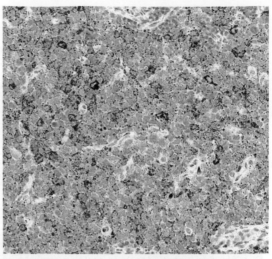

Fig. 5. Chromogranin A stains NE cells with a granular positivity of cytoplasm (original magnification ×20).

presence of associated endocrinopathies, or in asymptomatic patients with a fast-growing anterior mediastinal mass. Fine needle aspiration biopsy is to be avoided because of the risks of inadequate tissue sampling for differential diagnosis, and the possibility of false-negative results.

Histologic diagnosis is preferentially made through a tru-cut biopsy or parasternal anterior mediastinotomy (Chamberlain procedure) (**Fig. 7**). Using these techniques tissue sampling is sufficient for immunohistologic studies, and for a differential diagnosis with other mediastinal neoplasms, such as thymomas, thymic carcinomas, or lymphomas.

There is no official staging system for NETTs and most investigators rely on Masaoka and colleagues'[39] staging system used for thymomas, modified in 1994[40] (**Table 3**).

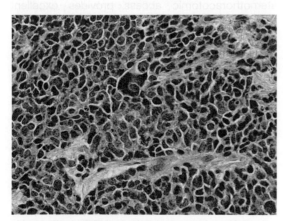

Fig. 4. Large-cell NE carcinoma showing marked cytologic atypias, scattered huge nuclei, and mitosis.

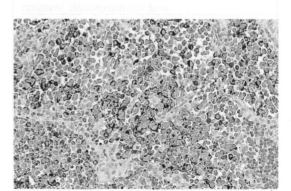

Fig. 6. Dotlike positivity of NE cells for cytokeratin AE1/AE3 (original magnification ×20).

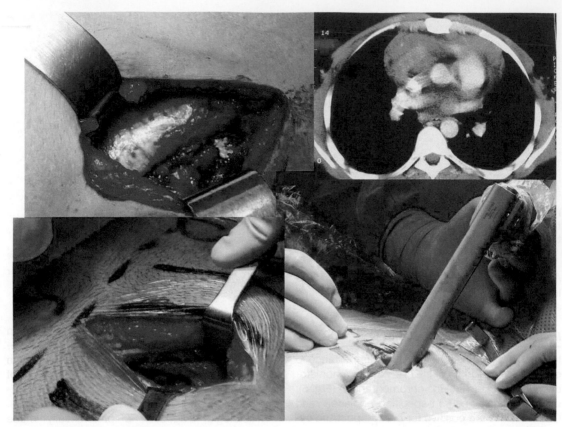

Fig. 7. Left anterior mediastinotomy (Chamberlain procedure) and mediastinoscopy: optimal surgical approach for a preoperative tissue biopsy in NETTs.

Table 4 shows the results of the most representative surgical series (>10 cases) of operated thymic NETTs published since 1990. Surgery is the mainstay of therapy even if large and locally invasive, because it provides dramatic symptom relief and a survival advantage over nonsurgical treatments.

Median sternotomy is the optimal surgical approach; anterior, lateral, or posterolateral thoracotomy may be used alone or in combination with sternotomy if the tumor extends laterally or if there is major invasion of the lungs; in this case, combined sternothoracotomic access provides excellent exposure.[41,42] Limited surgical approaches and minimally invasive techniques have no role in the treatment of NETTs.

Surgery should allow complete resection whenever possible, also in case of locally invasive tumors; the resectability rate among the published series ranges from 28% to 100% (mean 86%) depending on the experience of the center.[14] Incomplete resections mostly result from the highly aggressive behavior of NETTs, with possible residuals in the heart, trachea, aorta, and phrenic nerves.

In case of NETTs associated with MEN-1, Teh[28] recommends palliative debulking surgery both for symptom relief and to facilitate adjuvant treatment. Also, in these patients NETT is the main cause of death, and for this reason it has been

Table 3 Clinical staging of primary NETTs (Masaoka stage system)	
Stage I	Macroscopically encapsulated and no microscopic invasion
Stage II	Macroscopic invasion into surrounding fatty tissue of mediastinal pleura or microscopic invasion into capsule
Stage III	Macroscopic invasion into neighboring organ(s)
Stage IVa	Pleural or pericardial dissemination
Stage IVb	Lymphogenous or hematogenous metastasis

Data from Masaoka A, Monden Y, Nakahara K, et al. Follow-up study of thymoma with special reference to their clinical stages. Cancer 1981;48:2485–92.

Table 4
Comparison of results in the published surgical series (>10 patients) of NETTs (since 1990)

Author (Year)	No	Mean Age (y) (Range)	Sex (Male/Female)	Associated Disease	Complete Resection (Number) (%)	Incomplete Resection (Number) (%)	Histology	Postoperative Treatment	5-y Survival (Number) (%)	10-y Survival (Number) (%)
de Montpreville et al (1996)[9]	14	53 (35–71)	11/3	1 MEN-1; 1 VRD	4 (28.5)	10 (71.5)	14 AC	NA	4/13 (31%)	0/13 (0%)
Fukai et al (1999)[10]	15	51 (19–73)	10/5	2 CS; 1 MG	13 (86.7%)	2 (13.3)	1 TC; 9 AC; 5 SCC	5 RT; 1 CT + RT; 1 CT	5 (33%)	1 (7%)
Moran and Suster (2000)[3]	80	58 (16–100)	59/21	4 CS	NA	NA	29 TC; 36 AC; 15 SCC	NA	12/42 (28%)	4/42 (10%)
Gal et al (2001)[11]	10	52 (26–77)	7/3	3 CS; 1 MEN-1	9 (90%)	1 (10%)	2 TC; 6 AC; 2 SCC	3 CT+RT; 2 RT	NA	NA
Tiffet et al (2003)[13]	12	58 (35–78)	8/4	2 MEN-1; 1 CS	9 (75%)	3 (25%)	3 TC; 6 AC; 2 LCNC; 1 SCC	3 RT; 1 CT; 1 RT + CT	50%	NA
Cardillo et al (2009)[14]	19	49 (31–69)	14/5	5 CS	19 (100%)	0 (0%)	8 TC; 6 AC; 5 LCNC	8 RT	18 (91.6%)	13 (69.8%)

Abbreviations: AC, atypical carcinoid; CS, Cushing syndrome; LCNC, large-cell NE carcinoma; MG, myasthenia gravis; NA, not available; SCC, small-cell carcinoma; TC, typical carcinoid; VRD, von Recklinghausen disease.

suggested to remove the thymus at the time of the parathyroidectomy performed for associated hyperparathyroidism using the same cervical access.[28,43,44] This strategy has been shown to reduce recurrence of symptoms from any ectopic parathyroid located within the thymic tissue, and to reduce the risk of occurrence of NETTs later in life. In NETTs associated with Cushing syndrome, the rate of complete resection is high even if the tumor is usually large and locally invasive. de Perrot[12] collected 25 cases from the literature and found a total resection rate of 68% (17 patients).

About half of patients with NETTs have lymphnode metastases at the time of surgical resection, but this condition has not been found to be associated with a poor outcome.[8,10,11]

The role of chemotherapy (CT) and radiotherapy (RT) has not been established yet, because of the paucity of the clinical series and the lack of standardized schedules and radiation doses. CT and RT have been suggested in a preoperative (induction) or postoperative (adjuvant) setting. Fukai and colleagues[10] treated 2 patients with NETTs at Masaoka stage IVb with preoperative CT + RT (1 case) and CT only (1 case) followed by surgery; complete resection was accomplished in both patients, who eventually received postoperative RT. Cardillo and colleagues[14] in their recent series used preoperative CT (1 case) and CT + RT (1 case) in 2 patients with Masaoka stage III thymic large-cell NE carcinomas; both patients were completely resected and received postoperative adjuvant RT; at follow-up the patients remained alive and disease free 69 and 73 months after surgery. We[22] previously reported on a patient with a large and invasive moderately differentiated thymic NE carcinoma completely resected after induction CT (4 courses of cisplatin and etoposide), RT (total dose 42 Gy), and octreotide (20 mg every 28 days) followed by postoperative RT; the patient remained disease free for 40 months, when local recurrence was diagnosed. Dham and colleagues[45] recently published a case of atypical thymic carcinoid in which induction therapy with tyrosine kinase receptor inhibitor (Sunitinib) plus octreotide resulted in a significant tumor downsizing, allowing complete surgical resection; the patient was alive without recurrence 12 months after the operation. From the analysis of these scattered reports, therefore, we suggest that preoperative CT and RT may be safely used and result on some occasions in good response rates in preparation for surgery. Postoperatively, RT is recommended, especially in incomplete resections or when the tumor is at an advanced Masaoka stage, in those cases RT may contribute to reducing the risks of local relapses, although it

has been found to have little effect on long-term survival.[10,11] Postoperative CT is associated with limited response rate and significant toxicity[46,47]; at present there are no standardized schedules and any center should refer to its own experience. **Table 4** shows the adjuvant treatment schedules administered in the largest NETTs series published in the literature since 1990.

The expression of somatostatin receptors by NE tumors has prompted many investigators to investigate the use of somatostatin analogues (octreotide, lanreotide).[22,45] Octreotide alone or in combination with α-interferon has been used as adjuvant treatment in MEN-1 syndrome NETTs,[28,48–50] with conflicting results that currently cannot support their use as standard treatment. Despite pre- and/or postoperative CT/RT and the extent of surgical tumor resection, recurrences are common in patients with NETTs.

Similarly to thymoma, recurrence may be local (in the bed of the resected tumor), regional (intrathoracic, excluding recurrence into the lung), or distant (extrathoracic or intraparenchymal into the lung). Local or regional recurrence sites include the mediastinum, mediastinal lymph nodes, lung, major blood vessels, chest wall, and supraclavicular region. Distant recurrence includes metastases in the liver, stomach, brain, kidney, bones, and adrenal gland. **Table 5** shows recurrence rates (local and distant) and their treatment, if available, in the major series published in literature.

In cases of resectable recurrence redo surgery may be proposed.[6,13,14,17] Economopoulos[6] suggested that long-term survival can be achieved with an aggressive surgical resection of the recurrence. Tiffet and colleagues[13] reported a case of redo surgery (followed by RT) for a local relapse in a previously radically resected NETT (large-cell NE carcinoma); the patient was alive and disease free 35 months after the second surgery. Cardillo and colleagues[14] reported 2 patients who developed local recurrences 25 and 35 months after the first intervention who were successfully submitted to redo surgery (through midline resternotomy); in both patients a complete resection of the recurrence was obtained and the patients were alive and disease free at follow-up. Sakuragi and colleagues[51] published a case report about a patient with NETT who developed 4 locoregional recurrences, all of which were successfully resected. In the last resection the tumor invaded the right atrium and the superior vena cava, and surgery was performed through a resternotomy, using cardiopulmonary bypass.

A new radiobiologic treatment of local recurrences or distant metastases is radiolabeled octreotide, which has yielded tumor growth

Table 5
Recurrence rate and treatment in published reports (>10 patients) of NETTs (since 1990)

Author (Year)	No of Cases	Recurrence (%)	Postoperative Treatment	Treatment of Recurrence
de Montpreville et al (1996)[9]	14	3 loc (25); 7 dist (58.3)	NA	NA
Fukai et al (1999)[10]	15	0 loc; 10 dist (76.9)	6 adjuv RT; 4 no adjuv therapy	NA
Moran and Suster (2000)[3]	80	18 loc (22.5); 20 dist (25)	NA	NA
Gal et al (2001)[11]	10	8 dist (80)	3 adjuv RT + CT; 2 adjuv RT	NA
Tiffet et al (2003)[13]	12	1 loc (8.3); 3 distant (25); 6 loc + dist (50)	6 recurrences had no adjuv RT	1 RS + RT; 4 CT; 5 CT + RT
Cardillo et al (2009)[14]	19	2 loc (10.5); 0 dist	1 no adjuv RT; 1 adjuv RT	2 RS

Abbreviations: adjuv RT, adjuvant (postoperative) radiotherapy; adjuv RT + CT, adjuvant radiotherapy plus chemotherapy; dist, distant metastases; loc, local recurrence; NA, not available; RS, redo surgery; RS + RT, redo surgery plus radiotherapy.

regression in animal models in somatostatin receptor–positive NE tumors.[52] The radionuclide can also be substituted with a chemotherapeutic drug that can target thymic NE carcinoma cells: despite the intriguing biologic rationale, at present the efficacy of this treatment has not been proved in any clinical trial.

PROGNOSTIC FACTORS AND FOLLOW-UP

Despite its high biologic aggressiveness, intermediate-term survival in NETTs is fairly good, although most series report poor long-term survival. Survival is strictly related to the histologic tumor subtype, and the degree of cell differentiation, with the highest survival advantage for low-grade differentiated tumors, and the lowest survival in the poorly differentiated forms.[10,11,13,14] As in thymomas, a major prognostic factor is the Masaoka stage, which expresses the local tumor aggressiveness and extent of invasion. Prognosis is also dependent on the presence of associated endocrinopathies. Patients with NETTs and Cushing syndrome or MEN-1 syndrome have a 65% 5-year mortality[2] compared with a 35% mortality in patients with NETTs without paraneoplastic syndromes.

Analysis of the different prognostic indicators in NETTs was undertaken by several investigators[9–11,13,14] and, despite the limits of retrospective nonrandomized studies, a high histologic tumor differentiation, the extent of surgical resection, tumor unresectability, the high clinical stage at presentation, and the presence of metastases at the time of diagnosis were all associated with decreased survival. Postoperative RT/CT seems to reduce the risk of local relapse, although with no effect on long-term survival. **Table 4** shows 5- and 10-year survival rates (when available) in the major NETT series.

Because of the high risk of tumor relapse or distant metastases, close follow-up is mandatory in any patient operated on for NETTs. Patients should be strictly followed up for up to 10 years. A thoracic computed tomography scan is the recommended imaging technique for follow-up; in suspected tumor recurrence, thoracic MRI and/or Octreoscan may be indicated to assess recurrence resectability.

SUMMARY

NETTs are rare and biologically highly aggressive mediastinal tumors, more frequent in males and sometimes associated with endocrinopathies (more frequently Cushing and MEN-1 syndromes). Surgery is the mainstay of the treatment, and it should be proposed whenever possible even in locally advanced tumors. Postoperative RT (alone or in association with CT) seems to reduce the risk of local tumor recurrence, although at present, both CT and RT are ineffective in prolonging long-term survival. Biologic treatment with somatostatin analogues (eg, octreotide or

lanreotide) before or after surgery have been anec-
dotally proposed, and at present there are no
ongoing clinical trials about these drugs. After
surgery, recurrences are common, either local or
distant; surgery, when feasible, may be proposed
for local relapses. Prognostic factors that have
been shown to negatively influence long-term
survival include histologic tumor differentiation
grade, the Masaoka stage at presentation, the
presence of associated endocrinopathy, the presence of metastases at the time of diagnosis, the
extent of surgical resection, and an incomplete
resection.

REFERENCES

1. Rosai J, Higa E. Mediastinal endocrine neoplasm of
   probable thymic origin related to carcinoid tumor.
   Cancer 1972;29:1061–74.
2. Wick MR, Scott RE, Li CY, et al. Carcinoid tumor of
   the thymus: a clinicopathologic report of seven
   cases with a review of the literature. Mayo Clin
   Proc 1980;55:246–54.
3. Moran CA, Suster S. Neuroendocrine carcinomas
   (carcinoid tumor) of the thymus: a clinicopathologic
   analysis of 80 cases. Am J Clin Pathol 2000;114:
   100–10.
4. Oberg K, Jelic S. Neuroendocrine bronchial and
   thymic tumors: ESMO clinical recommendation for
   diagnosis, treatment and follow-up. Ann Oncol
   2008;19:ii102–3.
5. Wick MR, Scheithauer BW, Weiland LH, et al.
   Primary mediastinal carcinoid tumors. Am J Surg
   Pathol 1982;6:195–205.
6. Economopoulos GC, Lewis JW, Lee MW, et al. Carcinoid tumors of the thymus. Ann Thorac Surg 1990;
   50:58–61.
7. Valli M, Fabris GA, Dewar A, et al. Atypical carcinoid
   tumour of the thymus: a study of eight cases. Histopathology 1994;24:371–5.
8. Wang DY, Chang DB, Kuo SH, et al. Carcinoid
   tumours of the thymus. Thorax 1994;49:357–60.
9. de Montpreville VT, Macchiarini P, Dulmet E. Thymic
   neuroendocrine carcinoma (carcinoid): a clinicopathologic study of fourteen cases. J Thorac Cardiovasc Surg 1996;111:134–41.
10. Fukai I, Masaoka A, Fujii Y, et al. Thymic neuroendo-
    crine tumor (thymic carcinoid): a clinicopathologic
    study in 15 patients. Ann Thorac Surg 1999;67:
    208–11.
11. Gal AA, Kornstein MJ, Cohen C. Neuroendocrine
    tumors of the thymus: a clinicopathologic and prog-
    nostic study. Ann Thorac Surg 2001;72:1179–82.
12. de Perrot M, Spiliopoulos A, Fisher S, et al. Neuroen-
    docrine carcinoma (carcinoid) of the thymus associ-
    ated with Cushing's syndrome. Ann Thorac Surg
    2002;73:675–81.
13. Tiffet O, Nicholson AG, Ladas G, et al. A clinico-
    pathologic study of 12 neuroendocrine tumors arising
    in the thymus. Chest 2003;124:141–6.
14. Cardillo G, Treggiari S, Paul MA, et al. Primary
    neuroendocrine tumours of the thymus: a clinico-
    pathologic and prognostic study in 19 patients. Eur
    J Cardiothorac Surg 2010;37:814–8.
15. Klemm KM, Moran CA. Primary neuroendocrine
    carcinomas of the thymus. Semin Diagn Pathol
    1999;16:32–41.
16. Verley JM, Hollmann KH. Tumours of the medias-
    tinum. In: Gresham GA, editor. Current histopa-
    thology, vol. 19. London: Kluwer Academic; 1992.
    p. 102–8.
17. Chaer R, Massad MG, Evans A, et al. Primary neuro-
    endocrine tumors of the thymus. Ann Thorac Surg
    2002;74:1733–40.
18. Van Brandt V, Heymann S, Van Marck E, et al. Atyp-
    ical presentation of an atypical carcinoid. Ann
    Thorac Surg 2009;88:2004–6.
19. John L, Hornick P, Lang S, et al. Giant thymic carci-
    noid. Postgrad Med J 1991;67:462–5.
20. Dusmet ME, McKneally MF. Pulmonary and thymic
    carcinoid tumors. World J Surg 1996;20:189–95.
21. Rosado de Christenson ML, Abbott GF, Kirejczky WM.
    Thoracic carcinoids: radiologic-pathologic correla-
    tions. Radiographics 1999;19:707–11.
22. Filosso PL, Actis dato GM, Ruffini E, et al. Multidisci-
    plinary treatment of advanced thymic neuroendo-
    crine carcinoma (carcinoid): report of a successful
    case and review of the literature. J Thorac Cardio-
    vasc Surg 2004;127:1215–9.
23. Lastoria S, Vergara E, Palmieri G, et al. In vivo detec-
    tion of malignant thymic masses by Indium-111-
    DTPA-D-pentetreotide scintigraphy. J Nucl Med
    1998;39:634–9.
24. Cadigan DG, Hollett PD, Collingwood PW, et al.
    Imaging of mediastinal thymic carcinoid tumor with
    radiolabelled somatostatin analogue. Clin Nucl
    Med 1996;21:487–8.
25. Groves AM, Mohan HK, Wegner EA, et al. Positron
    emission tomography with FDG to show thymic
    carcinoid. AJR Am J Roentgenol 2004;182:511–3.
26. Duh QY, Hybarger CP, Geist R, et al. Carcinoids
    associated with multiple endocrine neoplasia
    syndromes. Am J Surg 1987;154:142–58.
27. Arrigoni MG, Woolner LB, Bernatz PE. Atypical
    carcinoid tumors of the lung. J Thorac Cardiovasc
    Surg 1972;64:413–21.
28. Teh BT. Thymic carcinoid tumors in multiple endocrine
    neoplasia type 1. J Intern Med 1998;243:501–4.
29. Levine GD, Rosai J. Thymic hyperplasia and
    neoplasia. A review of current concepts. Hum Pathol
    1978;9:295–514.
30. Marchevsky AM, Dikman SH. Mediastinal carcinoid
    with an incomplete Sipple's syndrome. Cancer
    1979;43:2497 501.

31. Wick MR, Rosai J. Neuroendocrine neoplasms of the thymus. Pathol Res Pract 1988;183:188–99.

32. Lowenthal RM, Gumpel JM, Kreel L, et al. Carcinoid tumor of the thymus with systemic manifestations: a radiological and pathological study. Thorax 1974; 92:553–8.

33. Wu MH;Tseng YL, Cheng FF, Lin TS. Thymic carcinoid combined with myasthenia gravis. J Thorac Cardiovasc Surg 2004;127:584–5.

34. Liu HC, Hsu WH, Chen YJ, et al. Primary thymic carcinoma. Ann Thorac Surg 2002;73:1076–81.

35. Marx A, Shimosato Y, Kuo TT, et al. Thymic neuroendocrine tumours. In: Travis WD, Brambilla E, Muller-Hermelink HK, et al, editors. WHO classification of tumours. Pathology and genetics of tumours of the lung, pleura, thymus and heart. Lyon (France): IARC Press; 2004. p. 188–95.

36. Suster S, Moran CA. Neuroendocrine neoplasms of the mediastinum. Am J Clin Pathol 2001;115(Suppl): S17–27.

37. Moran CA. Primary neuroendocrine carcinomas of the mediastinum: review of current criteria for histopathologic diagnosis and classification. Semin Diagn Pathol 2005;22(3):223–9.

38. Wakely PE Jr. Cytopathology-histopathology of the mediastinum II. Mesenchymal, neural, and neuroendocrine neoplasms. Ann Diagn Pathol 2005;9(1):24–32.

39. Masaoka A, Monden Y, Nakahara K, et al. Follow-up study of thymoma with special reference to their clinical stages. Cancer 1981;48:2485–92.

40. Koga K, Matsuno Y, Noguchi M, et al. A review of 79 thymomas: modification of staging system and reappraisal of conventional division into invasive and non-invasive thymoma. Pathol Int 1994;44(5):359–67.

41. Huang J, Riely GJ, Rosenzweig KE, et al. Multimodality therapy for locally invasive thymomas: state of the art or investigational therapy? Ann Thorac Surg 2008;85:365–7.

42. Huang J, Rizk NP, Travis WD, et al. Feasibility of multimodality therapy including extended resections in stage IVA thymoma. J Thorac Cardiovasc Surg 2007;134:1477–84.

43. Zeiger MA, Swartz SE, MacGillivray DC, et al. Thymic carcinoid in association with MEN syndromes. Am J Surg 1992;58:430–4.

44. Trump D, Farren B, Wooding C, et al. Clinical studies of multiple endocrine neoplasia type 1 (MEN-1). QJM 1996;89:653–69.

45. Dham A, Truskinovsky AM, Dudek AZ. Thymic carcinoid responds to neoadjuvant therapy with sunitinib and octreotide: a case report. J Thorac Oncol 2008; 3:94–7.

46. Hage R, de la Rivière AB, Seldenrijk CA, et al. Update in pulmonary carcinoid tumors. A review article. Ann Surg Oncol 2003;10:697–704.

47. Kosmidis PA. Treatment of carcinoid of the lung. Curr Opin Oncol 2004;16:146–9.

48. Oberg K, Norheim I, Theodorsson E. Treatment of malignant midgut carcinoid tumors with a long acting somatostatin analogue octreotide. Acta Oncol 1991;30:503–7.

49. Teh BT, McArdle J, Chan SP, et al. Clinicopathologic studies of thymic carcinoids in multiple endocrine neoplasia type 1. Medicine 1997;76:21–9.

50. Ferolla P, Falchetti A, Filosso PL, et al. Thymic neuroendocrine carcinoma (carcinoid) in multiple endocrine neoplasia type 1 syndrome: the Italian series. J Clin Endocrinol Metab 2005;90:2603–9.

51. Sakuragi T, Rikitake K, Nastuaki M, et al. Complete resection of recurrent thymic carcinoid using cardiopulmonary bypass. Eur J Cardiothorac Surg 2002; 21:152–4.

52. Slooter GD, Breenan WA, Marqnet RL, et al. Antiproliferative effect of radiolabeled octreotide in a metastases model in rat liver. Int J Cancer 1999; 81:767–71.

Thymic Carcinoma: Is it a Separate Entity? From Molecular to Clinical Evidence

Alexander Marx, MD[a],*, Ralf Rieker, MD[b,c],
Alper Toker, MD[d], Florian Länger, MD[e], Philipp Ströbel, MD[a]

KEYWORDS
• Thymic carcinomas • Thymomas
• Thymic squamous cell carcinomas

Thymic carcinomas (TCs) are rare tumors of the mediastinum. Their exact incidence is not known but can be estimated to be around 1 to 3 cases per 10 million inhabitants.[1–8] Due to unfortunate choices and changes in terminology, there has been considerable confusion about the biology and clinical behavior of these tumors. The current (2004) edition of the World Health Organization (WHO) classification[9] of thymic tumors separates TCs from thymomas for good reasons; thymomas are organotypic tumors (ie, their morphology is unique and not found in tumors of other organs, and they exhibit functional features of a normal thymus). The hallmark of such an organotypic function is the generation of immature T cells by the neoplastic epithelium. By contrast, thymic carcinomas are nonorganotypic tumors (ie, similar tumors are also encountered in many other organs [eg, head and neck or lung], and they do not have the capacity to promote the maturation of intratumorous immature T cells). In the past, much confusion was created by the introduction of the term "well differentiated thymic carcinoma".[10] It is now clear that these tumors are actually thymomas[11] (because they generate immature T cells), and they are now listed as type B3 thymomas in the WHO classification.[9]

Another critical issue related to TCs is to appreciate the fact that TC per se is not a proper diagnosis (as sarcoma does not denote a single entity, but rather a group of very different tumors) and tumors must be further subclassified into squamous cell, neuroendocrine, basaloid, lymphoepithelioma-like, clear cell carcinomas of the thymus, and many others. Although clinical data are scarce for most of these subtypes, the existing data show that it is not appropriate to list TCs without further reference to their subtype as a single group (eg, in studies dealing with clinical outcome). Many of the controversies in the literature about the prognosis and other critical features of TCs are due to such inconsistencies in terminology. This article will summarize the current knowledge on biologic and therapeutic aspects of thymic carcinomas with emphasis on the different histologic subtypes.

This work was supported by grant # 10-1740 from the Deutsche Krebshilfe and by Project grant 781025 of the Tumorzentrum Heidelberg/Mannheim.
a Institute of Pathology, University Medical Center Mannheim, University of Heidelberg, Theodor-Kutzer-Ufer 1-3, D-68135 Mannheim, Germany
b Institute of Pathology, University of Erlangen, Krankenhausstrasse 22, D91054 Erlangen, Germany
c Institute for Pathology, University Hospital, Heidelberg, Germany
d Thoracic Surgery, Istanbul University, 34093 Capa-Istanbul, Turkey
e Thoracic Surgery, Institute of Pathology, Medizinische Hochschule Hannover, Carl-Neuberg-strasse 1, D-30625 Hannover, Germany
* Corresponding author.
E-mail address: alexander.marx@umm.de

Thorac Surg Clin 21 (2011) 25–31
doi:10.1016/j.thorsurg.2010.08.010
1547-4127/11/$ — see front matter © 2011 Elsevier Inc. All rights reserved.

EPIDEMIOLOGY AND PROGNOSIS OF THE THYMIC CARCINOMA SUBTYPES LISTED IN THE WHO CLASSIFICATION

The WHO classification of 2004 recognizes 11 subtypes: squamous cell, basaloid, mucoepidermoid, lymphoepithelioma-like, sarcomatoid, clear cell, papillary and nonpapillary adenocarcinomas, carcinoma with t(15;19) translocation, undifferentiated carcinoma, and neuroendocrine tumors (carcinoid, atypical carcinoid, and small and large cell neuroendocrine carcinomas). Of these, however, only squamous cell carcinomas (TSCCs), lymphoepithelioma-like carcinomas, and the neuroendocrine tumors are more common (**Table 1, Fig. 1**). TSCCs account for up to 40% (27%–60%),[12–16] lymphoepithelioma-like carcinomas account for 15% (5%– 32%), neuroendocrine tumors for 18% (10%–30%) of cases. Most (15%) of the remaining cases consist of undifferentiated carcinomas.

Correct distinction between these entities is important, because the prognosis of TSCC is considerably better than that of the other carcinoma types.[13,15–17] In fact, many studies[5,6,18–20] found the prognosis of TSCC to be similar to type B3 thymoma with 10-year survival rates of 45%–65%.[5,6,15,20] Among the remaining types, a relatively favorable prognosis also has been reported for well differentiated neuroendocrine tumors (typical and atypical carcinoids), with reported 5-year survival rates between 28% and 75%.[21–23] A more favorable prognosis initially also was attributed to basaloid carcinomas, but this traditional view has recently been challenged.[24] Prognosis is now thought resemble that of other aggressive entities, with a median survival of 20 to 34 months.[13,15–17] Of note, the highly aggressive "carcinoma with t(15;19) translocation" has now been recognized as a midline carcinoma[25] that occurs in the upper aerodigestive tract, mediastinum, and abdomen and most likely is not a thymus derivative.

Clinical Presentation and Staging of Thymic Carcinomas

Symptomatic patients present with dull chest pain, cough, or dyspnea and constitutional symptoms. Superior vena cava syndrome is seen in patients with more advanced tumors. Paraneoplastic myasthenia gravis, the hallmark autoimmune manifestation of thymomas, is not seen in patients with TCs. Rarely, TCs are associated with polymyositis or dermatomyositis[26–29] or erythrocytosis caused by erythropoetin production.[30]

Neuroendocrine tumors may be associated with Cushing syndrome, while carcinoid syndrome is rare.[2] Neuroendocrine tumors of presumptive thymic origin also have been reported to occur in association with multiple endocrine neoplasia syndrome 1 (MEN-1).[23,31–33]

There is currently no authorized TNM staging system for thymic epithelial and neuroendocrine tumors. It is important to note that there seem to be major biologic differences between thymomas and TCs. Lymph node metastasis is exceedingly rare in thymomas, but is not unusual in thymic carcinomas, especially in neuroendocrine variants.

Therefore, the Masaoka staging system, which is widely used for thymomas (and which does not list lymph node metastasis as a separate staging criterion) appears suboptimal for TCs. In the current WHO volume on tumors of the thymus,[9] a tentative classification of malignant thymic epithelial tumors (thymomas and TCs including neuroendocrine tumors) was listed. It is mainly based on the Masaoka system and its revised versions.[34–36] However, the clinical feasibility of the listed lymph node stages has not been tested in larger case collections and awaits further investigation. Besides lymph nodes,

---

Table 1
Distribution of histologic subtypes of thymic carcinomas in published series

	TSCC (%)	LELC (%)	NEC (%)	UTC (%)	Other (%)
Chalabreysse et al[12]	29	12	23	6	30
Chen et al[5]	60	10	16	12	2
Dorfman et al[14]	38	17	30	8	7
Hsu et al[13]	40	5	10	35	10
Kuo et al[16]	46	15	15	NA	24
Suster & Rosai[15]	27	32	13	12	16

Abbreviations: LELC, lymphoepithelioma-like carcinoma; NA, not available; NEC, neuroendocrine carcinoma (including carcinoids, atypical carcinoids, large and small cell neuroendocrine carcinomas); TSCC, thymic squamous cell carcinoma; UTC, undifferentiated thymic carcinoma.

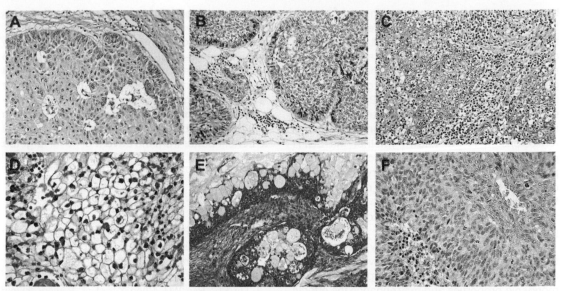

Fig. 1. Histologic appearance of some of the most frequent subtypes of thymic carcinomas. (*A*) Squamous cell carcinoma. (*B*) Basaloid carcinoma. (*C*) Lymphoepithelioma-like carcinoma. (*D*) Clear cell carcinoma. (*E*) Mucoepidermoid carcinoma. (*F*) Large cell neuroendocrine carcinoma. (*From* Rosai J, Sobin LH. World Health Organization histological classification of tumours. Histological typing of tumours of the thymus. 2nd edition. Berlin-Heidelberg (Germany): Springer-Verlag; 1999; with kind permission from Springer Science and Business Media.)

metastatic spread also involves cavitary dissemination in the pleural space and distant hematogenous metastases to lung, bone, and liver.

BASIC THERAPEUTIC APPROACHES IN THYMIC CARCINOMAS

The optimal treatment of thymic carcinoma remains an open issue and is beyond the scope of this article.[37–46] Similar to malignant thymomas, complete surgical excision, whenever possible, is the treatment of choice for early stage TCs and is prognostically important.[6,47] Most patients, however, present in advanced tumor stages, with evidence of invasion of adjacent mediastinal structures in approximately 80% of cases and radiologically apparent lymphadenopathy in approximately 40%.[48,49] In such cases, aggressive multimodal therapy with surgical resection, platinum-based combination chemotherapy, and radiotherapy is the therapeutic approach preferred by many authors.[38–43] For borderline or clearly unresectable cases, neoadjuvant chemotherapy with or without radiotherapy is applied.[44–46]

The Molecular Biology of Thymic Carcinomas and Implications for So-called Targeted Treatments

Genetic analyses are so far available only for TSCCs.[50–52] Single case descriptions on the cytogenetics of TCs suggest that the karyotype may be complex and hyperploid.[53] By conventional and array comparative genomic hybridization (CGH), TSCCs show recurrent genomic alterations, namely losses of chromosomes 1q, 6q, 13q, and gains of chromosome 1q, 17q, and 18. Interestingly, and in agreement with their similar prognosis, the genetic alterations found in TSCC and B3 thymomas show significant overlap and are clearly different from squamous cell carcinomas of the lung or head and neck.[52,54]

There are very few data on mutations of classical tumor suppressor genes or oncogenes. TP53 overexpression has been observed in most of TCs by immunohistochemistry,[55–57] and TP53 gene mutations can be detected in 30% of TCs.[57] TSCCs but not neuroendocrine carcinomas have been shown to frequently express FOXN1,[58] a transcription factor important for thymic organogenesis and, if deleted, responsible for the nude phenotype in mice.[59] This finding is interesting, because it raises the possibility that thymic carcinomas may be derived from a thymic epithelial progenitor cell.

Some studies analyzed the expression and mutation status of receptor tyrosine kinases. The epidermal growth factor receptor (EGFR) is strongly expressed in most thymomas,[60–63] and also in about 35% of thymic carcinomas.[63] There has also been evidence that the *EGFR* gene may be amplified in some thymic carcinomas.[62] Mutations of the EGFR and of downstream molecules that could interfere with EGFR antagonists, such as *KRAS/HRAS* or *BRAF*, are exceedingly rare.[52,63–66] In spite of initial observations suggesting effectiveness of EGFR targeting in some patients,[67–69] two clinical phase 2 studies using erlotinib[67] and gefitinib[70] in 44 patients resulted in no complete remission and only two partial remissions. It is not known whether the *EGFR* gene amplification status influences the therapeutic response rate. In summary, the existing data have been disappointing and do not suggest that targeting the EGFR in patients with TCs (and also malignant thymomas) is able to control tumor growth and progression.

There is evidence that the new generation of cyclooxygenase-2 (COX-2) selective nonsteroidal anti-inflammatory drugs (NSAIDs) possess antitumorigenic properties and may enhance the effects of EGFR inhibitors.[71] Cyclooxygenases catalyze the enzymatic conversion of arachidonic acid to prostaglandins and represent specific targets of NSAIDs. COX-2 is inducible, and increased concentrations have been observed in inflamed and tumorous tissue.[72] Most thymomas and TCs show increased expression of COX-2,[73] and application of a selective COX-2 inhibitor reduced cell viability in a TC cell line in vitro.[53]

Another consistent feature of TCs is strong expression of c-KIT (CD117), which is found in 75% to 100% of TSCCs[60,74,75] and also in most basaloid TCs.[24] However, mutations of *c-KIT* are rare and found in only up to 5% to 10% of cases.[52,63,64,75] The published mutations were located in exon 11 (delV560, L576P),[52,64,76] exon 14 (H697Y),[52] and exon17 (D820E).[77] These findings are of clinical relevance, because they suggest that imatinib may be a therapeutic option in TCs with KIT mutations,[76] while nonmutated tumors are refractory to this treatment.[78,79] Girard and colleagues[52] found that the H697Y mutation in exon 14 of *KIT* confers sensitivity to sunitinib. A recently published small series of four patients with advanced chemorefractory TCs suggested that sunitinib may be a promising treatment option in a subset of patients.[80] The findings in this series (all wild-type for KIT including exon 14) suggest that the presence of a KIT mutation may not be a prerequisite for clinical response.

SUMMARY

TC is a designation for a heterogeneous group of rare tumors. The distinction from thymomas and the exact definition of the histologic subtype (eg, squamous cell vs mucoepidermoid vs neuroendocrine) has important implications for both prognosis and therapy. In spite of a considerable body of data (mostly retrospective), there remain many open questions with regard to staging and the optimal choice of stage-adopted therapy. There is clearly a need to improve the results of current adjuvant and neoadjuvant strategies, but also more information about the genetics and molecular biology of these tumors is required to benefit better from the advent of novel targeted approaches.

REFERENCES

1. Engels EA, Pfeiffer RM. Malignant thymoma in the United States: demographic patterns in incidence and associations with subsequent malignancies. Int J Cancer 2003;105:546–51.
2. Liu HC, Hsu WH, Chen YJ, et al. Primary thymic carcinoma. Ann Thorac Surg 2002;73:1076–81.
3. Okumura M, Miyoshi S, Fujii Y, et al. Clinical and functional significance of WHO classification on human thymic epithelial neoplasms: a study of 146 consecutive tumors. Am J Surg Pathol 2001;25: 103–10.
4. Kim BK, Cho BC, Choi HJ, et al. A single institutional experience of surgically resected thymic epithelial tumors over 10 years: clinical outcomes and clinicopathologic features. Oncol Rep 2008; 19:1525–31.
5. Chen G, Marx A, Wen-Hu C, et al. New WHO histologic classification predicts prognosis of thymic epithelial tumors: a clinicopathologic study of 200 thymoma cases from China. Cancer 2002;95:420–9.
6. Strobel P, Bauer A, Puppe B, et al. Tumor recurrence and survival in patients treated for thymomas and thymic squamous cell carcinomas: a retrospective analysis. J Clin Oncol 2004;22:1501–9.
7. Engel P, Marx A, Muller-Hermelink HK. Thymic tumours in Denmark. A retrospective study of 213 cases from 1970–1993. Pathol Res Pract 1999; 195:565–70.
8. Okereke IC, Kesler KA, Morad MH, et al. Prognostic indicators after surgery for thymoma. Ann Thorac Surg 2010;89:1071–7 [discussion: 1077–9].
9. Müller-Hermelink HK, Engel P, Kuto TT, et al. Tumours of the thymus: introduction. In: Travis MD, Brambilla E. Müller-Hermelink HK, et al, editors. World Health Organization classification of tumours. Pathology and genetics. Tumours of the lung, pleura, thymus and heart. Lyon (France): IARC Press; 2004. p.145–51.
10. Kirchner T, Schalke B, Buchwald J, et al. Well-differentiated thymic carcinoma. An organotypical low-grade carcinoma with relationship to cortical thymoma. Am J Surg Pathol 1992;16:1153–69.

11. Masaoka A, Yamakawa Y, Fujii Y. Well-differentiated thymic carcinoma: is it thymic carcinoma or not? J Thorac Cardiovasc Surg 1999;117:628–30.

12. Chalabreysse L, Roy P, Cordier JF, et al. Correlation of the WHO schema for the classification of thymic epithelial neoplasms with prognosis: a retrospective study of 90 tumors. Am J Surg Pathol 2002;26: 1605–11.

13. Hsu CP, Chen CY, Chen CL, et al. Thymic carcinoma. Ten years' experience in twenty patients. J Thorac Cardiovasc Surg 1994;107:615–20.

14. Dorfman DM, Shahsafaei A, Chan JK. Thymic carcinomas, but not thymomas and carcinomas of other sites, show CD5 immunoreactivity. Am J Surg Pathol 1997;21:936–40.

15. Suster S, Rosai J. Thymic carcinoma. A clinicopathologic study of 60 cases. Cancer 1991;67:1025–32.

16. Kuo TT, Chang JP, Lin FJ, et al. Thymic carcinomas: histopathological varieties and immunohistochemical study. Am J Surg Pathol 1990;14:24–34.

17. Wick MR, Scheithauer BW, Weiland LH, et al. Primary thymic carcinomas. Am J Surg Pathol 1982;6:613–30.

18. Rieker RJ, Hoegel J, Morresi-Hauf A, et al. Histologic classification of thymic epithelial tumors: comparison of established classification schemes. Int J Cancer 2002;98:900–6.

19. D'Angelillo RM, Trodella L, Ramella S, et al. Novel prognostic groups in thymic epithelial tumors: assessment of risk and therapeutic strategy selection. Int J Radiat Oncol Biol Phys 2008;71: 420–7.

20. Kondo K, Yoshizawa K, Tsuyuguchi M, et al. WHO histologic classification is a prognostic indicator in thymoma. Ann Thorac Surg 2004;77:1183–8.

21. Kondo K, Monden Y. Therapy for thymic epithelial tumors: a clinical study of 1320 patients from Japan. Ann Thorac Surg 2003;76:878–84 [discussion: 884–5].

22. Gal AA, Kornstein MJ, Cohen C, et al. Neuroendocrine tumors of the thymus: a clinicopathological and prognostic study. Ann Thorac Surg 2001;72: 1179–82.

23. Zeiger MA, Swartz SE, MacGillivray DC, et al. Thymic carcinoid in association with MEN syndromes. Am Surg 1992;58:430–4.

24. Brown JG, Familiari U, Papotti M, et al. Thymic basaloid carcinoma: a clinicopathologic study of 12 cases, with a general discussion of basaloid carcinoma and its relationship with adenoid cystic carcinoma. Am J Surg Pathol 2009;33:1113–24.

25. French CA, Kutok JL, Faquin WC, et al. Midline carcinoma of children and young adults with NUT rearrangement. J Clin Oncol 2004;22:4135–9.

26. Inoue Y, True LD, Martins RG. Thymic carcinoma associated with paraneoplastic polymyositis. J Clin Oncol 2009;27:e33–4.

27. Azuma Y, Shiga K, Ishii R, et al. Polymyositis with atypical pathological features associated with thymic carcinoma. Intern Med 2009;48:163–8.

28. Takahashi F, Tsuta K, Nagaoka T, et al. Successful resection of dermatomyositis associated with thymic carcinoma: report of a case. Surg Today 2008;38: 245–8.

29. Koppula BR, Pipavath S, Lewis DH. Epstein-Barr virus (EBV) associated lymphoepithelioma-like thymic carcinoma associated with paraneoplastic syndrome of polymyositis: a rare tumor with rare association. Clin Nucl Med 2009;34:686–8.

30. Munakata W, Ohashi K, Sakaguchi K, et al. Erythrocytosis caused by erythropoietin-producing thymic carcinoma. Int J Clin Oncol 2010;15:220–3.

31. Tiffet O, Nicholson AG, Ladas G, et al. A clinicopathologic study of 12 neuroendocrine tumors arising in the thymus. Chest 2003;124:141–6.

32. Moran CA, Suster S. Neuroendocrine carcinomas (carcinoid tumor) of the thymus. A clinicopathologic analysis of 80 cases. Am J Clin Pathol 2000;114: 100–10.

33. Wang DY, Chang DB, Kuo SH, et al. Carcinoid tumours of the thymus. Thorax 1994;49:357–60.

34. Masaoka A, Monden Y, Nakahara K, et al. Follow-up study of thymomas with special reference to their clinical stages. Cancer 1981;48:2485–92.

35. Tsuchiya R, Koga K, Matsuno Y, et al. Thymic carcinoma: proposal for pathological TNM and staging. Pathol Int 1994;44:505–12.

36. Yamakawa Y, Masaoka A, Hashimoto T, et al. A tentative tumor-node-metastasis classification of thymoma. Cancer 1991;68:1984–7.

37. Rajan A, Giaccone G. Treatment of advanced thymoma and thymic carcinoma. Curr Treat Options Oncol 2008;9:277–87.

38. Ogawa K, Toita T, Uno T, et al. Treatment and prognosis of thymic carcinoma: a retrospective analysis of 40 cases. Cancer 2002;94:3115–9.

39. Latz D, Schraube P, Oppitz U, et al. Invasive thymoma: treatment with postoperative radiation therapy. Radiology 1997;204:859–64.

40. Greene MA, Malias MA. Aggressive multimodality treatment of invasive thymic carcinoma. J Thorac Cardiovasc Surg 2003;125:434–6.

41. Loehrer PJ Sr. Current approaches to the treatment of thymoma. Ann Med 1999;2(Suppl 31):73–9.

42. Venuta F, Rendina EA, Longo F, et al. Long-term outcome after multimodality treatment for stage III thymic tumors. Ann Thorac Surg 2003;76:1866–72 [discussion: 1872].

43. Venuta F, Rendina EA, Coloni GF. Multimodality treatment of thymic tumors. Thorac Surg Clin 2009;19: 71–81.

44. Eng TY, Fuller CD, Jagirdar J, et al. Thymic carcinoma: state of the art review. Int J Radiat Oncol Biol Phys 2004;59:654–64.

45. Hsu HC, Huang EY, Wang CJ, et al. Postoperative radiotherapy in thymic carcinoma: treatment results and prognostic factors. Int J Radiat Oncol Biol Phys 2002;52:801–5.

46. Mayer R, Beham-Schmid C, Groell R, et al. Radiotherapy for invasive thymoma and thymic carcinoma. Clinicopathological review. Strahlenther Onkol 1999;175:271–8.

47. Lucchi M, Mussi A, Basolo F, et al. The multimodality treatment of thymic carcinoma. Eur J Cardiothorac Surg 2001;19:566–9.

48. Jung KJ, Lee KS, Han J, et al. Malignant thymic epithelial tumors: CT-pathologic correlation. AJR Am J Roentgenol 2001;176:433–9.

49. Lee JD, Choe KO, Kim SJ, et al. CT findings in primary thymic carcinoma. J Comput Assist Tomogr 1991;15:429–33.

50. Zettl A, Strobel P, Wagner K, et al. Recurrent genetic aberrations in thymoma and thymic carcinoma. Am J Pathol 2000;157:257–66.

51. Penzel R, Hoegel J, Schmitz W, et al. Clusters of chromosomal imbalances in thymic epithelial tumours are associated with the WHO classification and the staging system according to Masaoka. Int J Cancer 2003;105:494–8.

52. Girard N, Shen R, Guo T, et al. Comprehensive genomic analysis reveals clinically relevant molecular distinctions between thymic carcinomas and thymomas. Clin Cancer Res 2009; 15:6790–9.

53. Ehemann V, Kern MA, Breinig M, et al. Establishment, characterization and drug sensitivity testing in primary cultures of human thymoma and thymic carcinoma. Int J Cancer 2008;122:2719–25.

54. Müller-Hermelink HK, Strobel P, Zettl A, et al. Metastases to thymus and anterior mediastinum. In: Travis MD, Brambilla E. Müller-Hermelink HK, et al, editors. World Health Organization classification of tumours. Pathology and genetics. Tumours of the lung, pleura, thymus and heart. Lyon (France): IARC Press; 2004. p. 247.

55. Chen FF, Yan JJ, Jin YT, et al. Detection of bcl-2 and p53 in thymoma: expression of bcl-2 as a reliable marker of tumor aggressiveness. Hum Pathol 1996; 27:1089–92.

56. Hirabayashi H, Fujii Y, Sakaguchi M, et al. p16INK4, pRB, p53 and cyclin D1 expression and hypermethylation of CDKN2 gene in thymoma and thymic carcinoma. Int J Cancer 1997;73: 639–44.

57. Tateyama H, Eimoto T, Tada T, et al. p53 protein expression and p53 gene mutation in thymic epithelial tumors. An immunohistochemical and DNA sequencing study. Am J Clin Pathol 1995;104: 375–81.

58. Nonaka D, Henley JD, Chirihoga L, et al. Diagnostic utility of thymic epithelial markers CD205 (DEC205) and Foxn1 in thymic epithelial neoplasms. Am J Surg Pathol 2007;31:1038–44.

59. Bleul CC, Corbeaux T, Reuter A, et al. Formation of a functional thymus initiated by a postnatal epithelial progenitor cell. Nature 2006;441:992–6.

60. Henley JD, Cummings OW, Loehrer PJ Sr. Tyrosine kinase receptor expression in thymomas. J Cancer Res Clin Oncol 2004;130:222–4.

61. Henley JD, Koukoulis GK, Loehrer PJ Sr. Epidermal growth factor receptor expression in invasive thymoma. J Cancer Res Clin Oncol 2002;128:167–70.

62. Ionescu DN, Sasatomi E, Cieply K, et al. Protein expression and gene amplification of epidermal growth factor receptor in thymomas. Cancer 2005; 103:630–6.

63. Strobel P, Knop S, Einsele H, et al. Therapy-relevant mutations of receptor tyrosine kinases in malignant thymomas and thymic carcinomas: a therapeutic perspective. Verh Dtsch Ges Pathol 2007;91:177–86.

64. Yoh K, Nishiwaki Y, Ishii G, et al. Mutational status of EGFR and KIT in thymoma and thymic carcinoma. Lung Cancer 2008;62:316–20.

65. Meister M, Schirmacher P, Dienemann H, et al. Mutational status of the epidermal growth factor receptor (EGFR) gene in thymomas and thymic carcinomas. Cancer Lett 2007;248:186–91.

66. Strobel P, Bargou R, Wolff A, et al. Sunitinib in metastatic thymic carcinomas: laboratory findings and initial clinical experience. Br J Cancer 2010;103(2): 196–200.

67. Christodoulou C, Murray S, Dahabreh J, et al. Response of malignant thymoma to erlotinib. Ann Oncol 2008;19:1361–2.

68. Farina G, Garassino MC, Gambacorta M, et al. Response of thymoma to cetuximab. Lancet Oncol 2007;8:449–50.

69. Palmieri G, Marino M, Salvatore M, et al. Cetuximab is an active treatment of metastatic and chemorefractory thymoma. Front Biosci 2007;12:757–61.

70. Kurup A, Burns M, Dropcho S, et al. Phase II study of gefitinib treatment in advanced thymic malignancies. J Clin Oncol 2005;23(16S):7068.

71. Chen Z, Zhang X, Li M, et al. Simultaneously targeting epidermal growth factor receptor tyrosine kinase and cyclooxygenase-2, an efficient approach to inhibition of squamous cell carcinoma of the head and neck. Clin Cancer Res 2004;10:5930–9.

72. Fosslien E. Biochemistry of cyclooxygenase (COX)-2 inhibitors and molecular pathology of COX-2 in neoplasia. Crit Rev Clin Lab Sci 2000;37:431–502.

73. Rieker RJ, Joos S, Mechtersheimer G, et al. COX-2 upregulation in thymomas and thymic carcinomas. Int J Cancer 2006;119:2063–70.

74. Pan CC, Chen PC, Chiang H. KIT (CD117) is frequently overexpressed in thymic carcinomas but is absent in thymomas. J Pathol 2004;202: 375–81.

75. Tsuchida M, Umezu H, Hashimoto T, et al. Absence of gene mutations in KIT-positive thymic epithelial tumors. Lung Cancer 2008;62:321–5.

76. Strobel P, Hartmann M, Jakob A, et al. Thymic carcinoma with overexpression of mutated KIT and the response to imatinib. N Engl J Med 2004;350: 2625–6.

77. Bisagni G, Rossi G, Cavazza A, et al. Long lasting response to the multikinase inhibitor bay 43–9006 (Sorafenib) in a heavily pretreated metastatic thymic carcinoma. J Thorac Oncol 2009;4:773–5.

78. Giaccone G, Rajan A, Ruijter R, et al. Imatinib mesylate in patients with WHO B3 thymomas and thymic carcinomas. J Thorac Oncol 2009;4: 1270–3.

79. Salter J, Lewis D, Yiannoutsos C, et al. Imatinib for the treatment of thymic carcinoma. J Clin Oncol 2008;2615S:8116.

80. Strobel P, Bargou R, Wolff A, et al. Sunitinib in metastatic thymic carcinomas: laboratory findings and initial clinical experience. Br J Cancer 2010;103: 196–200.

Immunohistochemistry of Thymic Epithelial Tumors as a Tool in Translational Research

Mirella Marino, MD[a],*, Mauro Piantelli, MD[b]

KEYWORDS

- Thymoma • Biomarkers
- Vascular endothelial growth factor
- Vascular endothelial growth factor receptor
- Immunohistochemistry

THYMIC EPITHELIAL TUMORS: THE WORLD HEALTH ORGANIZATION CLASSIFICATION AND ITS PROGNOSTIC VALUE

Due to their heterogeneity and infrequency, thymic epithelial cell tumors (TET) represent a diagnostic as well as a therapeutic problem. An incidence rate of 1 to 5 cases per million individuals per year has been reported. The occurrence of malignant cases is around 1.5 per million individuals per year. In the early stage of disease TET are usually cured by performing radical resections, whereas in advanced stages of disease they are usually radically unresectable from the beginning, and often show multiple relapses and/or intra- or extrathoracic metastases. The World Health Organization (WHO) classification of TET in 1999 and 2004 (**Box 1**)[1] established a milestone in diagnostic pathology, allowing comparison of various previously established classifications (**Table 1**),[2,3] and later becoming the reference classification for most surgeons, clinicians, and researchers in thymic pathology. The WHO classification is essentially based on the histogenetic classification of TET[3]; it has gained wide acceptance and has been shown to be of prognostic value by several studies published in the last decade.[4–17] In TET diagnostics, the pathologic workup of thymic tumors is mainly based on the microscopic examination of formalin-fixed and paraffin-embedded tissue stained with the routine stain, namely, hematoxylin-eosin (H&E). Trained pathologists are required in TET diagnostics; awareness of the complexity of the mediastinum and of the differential diagnostic possibilities[18] is mandatory. There is as yet no unanimous agreement among pathologists in using the WHO classification[19–21]; another classification scheme has been proposed (**Table 2**).[22] However, recent data (presented at the 2009 European Society of Pathology Meeting in Florence, Italy) (Müller-Hermelink, Bei Huang, Marino and colleagues, unpublished results, 2009) highlighted the reliability and reproducibility of the 2004 WHO classification of TET. A widely used pathologic classification, however, is the first prerequisite in understanding inherent tumor biology and oncological properties.

The role of the pathologist has gradually changed over the last decade; nevertheless, histopathological criteria are still essential in aiding clinicians in

Disclosure: the authors declare no potential conflicts of interest.

This work was supported by grants from the US and Italian National Health Institutes (US-Italian NHI program for Rare Diseases, 2006). Part of the data were presented at the First International Thymic Malignancy Interest Group (ITMIG) Meeting held in New York, NY, USA, May 5–6, 2010.

[a] Department of Pathology, Regina Elena National Cancer Institute, Via Elio Chianesi 53, 00144 Rome, Italy

[b] Department of Oncology and Neurosciences, "G. D'Annunzio" University and Foundation Chieti-Pescara, Via dei Vestini 5, 66013 Chieti, Italy

* Corresponding author.

E-mail address: mirellamarino@inwind.it

Thorac Surg Clin 21 (2011) 33–46

doi:10.1016/j.thorsurg.2010.08.014

the management of cancer patients. Current pathology reports usually include the use of ancillary techniques such as immunohistochemistry (IHC) to define histopathological tumor variants and to provide prognostic as well as predictive information. Immunohistochemical studies play a fundamental role in oncologic surgical pathology. In fact IHC help to establish diagnosis in crushed specimens, in classifying tumors, in predicting the likely origin of carcinomas, in demonstrating micrometastases, and in providing prognostic information. Furthermore, IHC provides a direct link between protein expression and histologic features, which allows a precise cellular or subcellular location of the target protein. In addition, the differential expression of proteins in normal versus malignant tissues can be studied. Among the many uses of IHC in cancer research, studies on a possible association between biomarker expression and treatment outcomes dominate the clinical translational research applications. The purpose of this review is to report and discuss the role of IHC in diagnostic and translational research of TET.

ROLE OF IMMUNOHISTOCHEMISTRY IN TET DIAGNOSTICS AND RESEARCH

In TET, evaluation IHC plays a fundamental role in the diagnostics of mediastinal biopsies (MB) and in fine-needle biopsies (FNB).[18] In addition, the evaluation of TET IHC may provide:

1. An assessment of TET differentiation antigens to set up an immunohistochemical diagnostic profile and tumor subtype characteristics
2. Evidence of a histogenetic relationship among different disease entities
3. A tissue-base evaluation of factors involved in TET development and progression and/or prognosis
4. Relevant predictive information for therapeutic purposes.

Immunohistochemistry to Assess TET Differentiation–Associated Antigens

The characterization of the EC cytokeratin and of other EC markers in TET is still in progress; new markers have also been described recently.[23–26] A TET cytokeratin profile of diagnostic value in the differential diagnosis of mediastinal/pulmonary and pleural neoplasms was defined by a survey of the wide and complex literature.[27–29] Furthermore, the evidence of a histogenetic correlation of thymoma with cortical and/or medullary derivation by an immunohistochemical profile[30] has been the focus of an extensive debate, even though some immunohistochemical correlations have been described.[31,32] Chilosi and colleagues[33] described the occurrence of CD20 as an aberrant marker in spindle EC of "mixed" type thymomas; this marker was shown to stain "medullary" EC type in thymomas. A further diagnostic improvement was the identification of CD5[34–37] as a marker for the squamous thymic carcinoma, and of KIT (CD117), which stains most thymic carcinomas at variance with most epithelial neoplasms.[38,39] Morphology (**Fig. 1**), clinicopathologic features, and IHC (**Fig. 2**) contributed to the definition of TET subtypes and of new TET variants.[40–46] It appears that any type of immunohistochemical marker investigated should be related to the current histologic classifications in order to be diagnostically relevant.

Principal Achievements of IHC in Biomarker Research

Several articles deal with prognostic and/or predictive marker research in TET. Only a few of them are discussed here according to the marker family. In several studies, the limited number of

Table 1
Comparison of the 1999 WHO classification of TET (center) with the clinicopathological classification of Levine and Rosai (left) and the histologic (or histogenetic) European classification of TET (right)

		Histologic Classification of Thymic Epithelial Tumors[b]
Clinicopathological Classification (1975)[a]	WHO Type (1999)	European Histogenetic Classification (1985)
Benign thymoma		Organotypic TET
	A	Medullary thymoma
	AB	Mixed thymoma
Malignant thymomas, Category I	B1	Predominantly cortical (organoid) thymoma
	B2	Cortical thymoma
	B3	Well-differentiated thymic carcinoma
Malignant thymomas, Category II	C	Nonorganotypic TET

[a] *Data from* Levine GD, Rosai J. Thymic hyperplasia and neoplasia: a review of current concepts. Hum Pathol 1978;9:495.
[b] *Data from* Marino M, Müller-Hermelink HK. Thymoma and thymic carcinoma. Relation of thymoma epithelial cells to the cortical and medullary differentiation of thymus. Virchows Arch A Pathol Anat Histopathol 1985;407:119; Kirchner T, Schalke B, Buchwald J, et al. Well-differentiated thymic carcinoma. An organotypical low-grade carcinoma with relationship to cortical thymoma. Am J Surg Pathol 1992;16:1153.

cases evaluated suggests that analysis of large case series is necessary to obtain statistically relevant informations.

THE p53 FAMILY AND RELATED FACTORS

The p53 oncosuppressor transcription family has been the focus of extensive research because of its role as a protective gene against tumor

Table 2
Comparison of the Suster and Moran classification (1999) with the 2004 WHO classification

Suster-Moran[a]	WHO[b]
Thymoma	Type A
	Type AB
	Type B1
	Type B2
Atypical thymoma	Type B3
Thymic	Thymic
Carcinoma	Carcinoma

The principle of the Suster-Moran classification is that the determination of the cytologic degree of EC atypia and the identification of the organotypical features of thymic differentiation permit to distinguish 3 simple diagnostic categories: thymoma, atypical thymoma, and thymic carcinoma.
[a] *Data from* Suster S, Moran CA. Primary thymic epithelial neoplasms: spectrum of differentiation and histologic features. Semin Diagn Pathol 1999;16:2.
[b] *Data from* Travis WD. Pathology & genetics. Tumours of the lung, pleura, thymus and heart. Lyon: IARC Press; 2004.

development in its wild-type form. Its role in TET has been repeatedly investigated over the last 15 years, p53 being the most frequently immunostained nuclear protein in TET. Hayashi and colleagues[47] first correlated the p53 immunohistochemical expression to clinicopathological variables showing a higher p53 expression in malignant thymoma type I and II versus benign thymoma according to Levine and Rosai,[2] particularly in advanced stages with respect to the early stages. p53 alterations were suggested as an early event in thymoma development. Tateyama and colleagues[48] also found point mutations, even in low p53 expression cases. However, subsequent studies failed to demonstrate genetic alterations in the p53 gene.[49–51] The immunohistochemical p53 staining patterns were heterogeneously detected due to different antibody types (polyclonal vs monoclonal). Overall, the polyclonal antibody CM1 reactivity to p53 was found to be associated with stage, histologic subtype, and survival time,[51] suggesting a p53 alteration, but to be unrelated to the genetic changes so far analyzed. Hiroshima and colleagues[52] found that overexpression of p53 as determined by the monoclonal antibody was associated with a higher tumor proliferative activity and with the B3 and C histotypes. The cell-cycle regulatory proteins p53, p21, and p27 were synchronously evaluated in different clinical settings of the thymomas (encapsulated thymomas; recurrent thymomas). The integrated protein expression pattern correlated with stage, WHO histotype, disease-free survival, and local recurrence rate.[53–55] These studies demonstrated the relevance and the

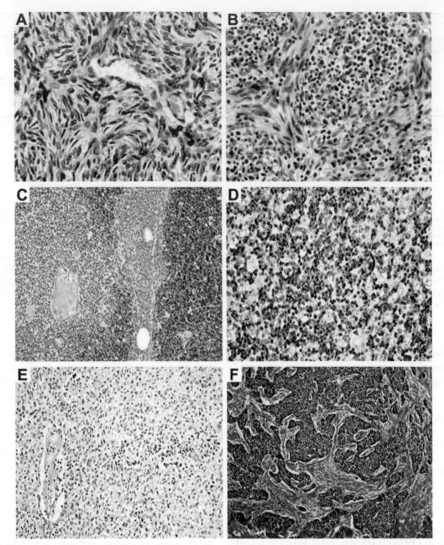

Fig. 1. TET subtypes as defined by the WHO 2004 classification. (*A*) Type A thymoma is defined as a spindle epithelial cell (EC) proliferation with absent or very few lymphocytes of mature T type (hematoxylin-eosin [H&E], original magnification ×400). (*B*) Type AB thymoma is defined as a combination of spindle EC areas with areas containing EC with dendritic morphology and large oval vesicular nucleus (H&E, original magnification ×200). (*C*) Type B1 thymoma is a rare lymphocyte-rich thymoma with EC with vesicular nucleus, forming cortex-like lobules and limited areas similar to thymic medulla (H&E, original magnification ×50). (*D*) Type B2 thymoma shows a higher EC content and an abundant lymphoid component of immature cortical thymocytes (H&E, original magnification ×200). (*E*) B3 thymoma is formed by EC arranged in sheets with minimal atypia forming perivascular spaces, with scant lymphoid content mostly of mature T cells (H&E, original magnification ×100). (*F*) A case of thymic carcinoma with sheets of cohesive, infiltrating EC, desmoplastic stroma, and absent lymphocytes. Squamous cell carcinoma is the most frequent subtype of thymic carcinoma (H&E, original magnification ×50).

interrelationship of the expression of the cell cycle regulatory check point proteins high p53, low p21, and low p27, which were related to a shorter disease-free survival[55] or recurrence.[54] The combined expression of p53 and Src, the nonreceptor protein kinase marker, was found by Khoury and colleagues[56] to be statistically significant, and their positive association was correlated with a shorter overall survival. Their study could not be sustained by a multivariate analysis due to the limited number of cases.

Other p53 Gene Family Members: p63

p63, a gene of the p53 gene family, is related to normal tissue development, survival, and

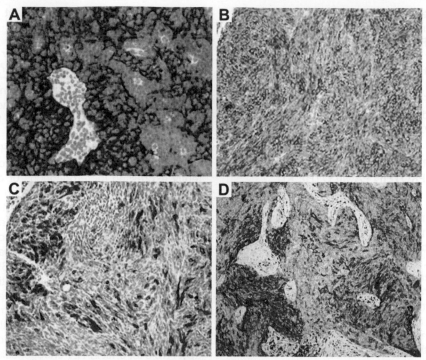

Fig. 2. Examples of IHC staining of TET. Immunohistochemical staining by cytokeratin 19 (CK19) (*A*) (original magnification ×200) and by the cocktail of cytokeratins MNF116 (CK MNF116) (*B*) (original magnification ×100) of a B2 and an A type thymoma, respectively. In (*C*) the stain of EC with CD20 in an A type thymoma is shown (original magnification ×100). (*D*) CD5 stain in a thymic carcinoma (original magnification ×100).

differentiation of stem cells, and it is expressed in stratified epithelia as well as by basal cells in glandular tissue (breast, prostate). p63 nuclear staining was described in thymomas[57] containing all the p63 isoforms. Subsequently,[58] among the p63 isoforms, ΔNp63α was clearly found in all the EC compartments of the normal thymus gland as well as in all thymomas, highlighting p63 constitutive expression and possibly relating all thymomas to a common thymic epithelial progenitor. By using primary cultures of thymic epithelial cells (TEC), p63 was shown to up-regulate the intercellular adhesion molecule-1 (ICAM-1), as well as interleukin (IL)-6 and IL-8 production. In vivo immunohistochemical staining demonstrated that p63 is found in all types of TEC, whereas p73, another epitheliotropic member of the p53 gene family, was found only in subcapsular and medullary TEC, highlighting the possibility of a new marker to distinguish between TEC subpopulations.[59] Among the apoptosis inhibitors, XIAP (X-linked inhibitor of apoptosis inhibitor) was found to be negative in the normal thymus tissue even though expressed in almost all thymomas. However, no correlation was found between encapsulated versus invasive TET in the 12 cases tested so far.[60]

OTHER APOPTOSIS-RELATED MARKERS

Among the apoptosis inhibitors, the bcl-2 proto-oncogene was evaluated in TET in association with the Mcl-1 protein, another member of the bcl-2 protein family, and with the apoptotic markers BAX, Bcl-XL, and cyclin-D1. Chen and colleagues[61] showed an inverse relationship between Mcl-1 and Bcl-2 expression, Mcl-1 being typically and closely associated with thymic carcinomas, and poorly expressed in thymoma and B3 tumors (well-differentiated thymic carcinoma).[40] In thymic carcinomas bcl-2 reactivity was seen in the less differentiated cells. The investigators speculated about the different roles played by these oncoproteins in the diverse types (thymic carcinoma and thymoma) of proliferations.

Among the apoptotic and oncogene markers, Pan and colleagues[62] found a high expression of Bcl-2 in thymic carcinomas, regardless of the histologic subtype, whereas thymomas showed a weak or no expression at all. These investigators suggested Bcl-2 and p53 to be implicated in the development of thymic carcinomas, and proposed these proteins as markers of aggression and predictors of nonresectability. An interesting approach was used by Salakou and colleagues,[63] who by means of IHC, mRNA in situ hybridization, and a TUNEL stain for apoptotic cells demonstrated that the Bax/Bcl-2 mRNA and protein ratios were higher in advanced stages, and were associated to caspase-3 expression and apoptosis. Furthermore, the Bax/Bcl-2 ratio was an independent prognostic factor of efficacy of thymectomy.

THE EPIDERMAL GROWTH FACTOR RECEPTOR PROTEIN FAMILY/THE KIT PROTEIN

The epidermal growth factor receptor (EGFR) family was investigated as far as its in situ expression is concerned by IHC in TET using several approaches. EGFR immunohistochemical detection has been reported in TET since 1993 by Pescarmona and colleagues[64] The expression of epidermal growth factor (EGF) and nerve growth factor (NGF) receptors were investigated by immunohistochemical analysis in 8 normal thymuses and in 15 thymomas. In normal thymuses, the EGFR was expressed by subcapsular, cortical, and medullary epithelial cells. In thymomas, irrespective of their histologic type, the EGFR, detected by a polyclonal antibody, was expressed by a large majority of EC. The investigators suggested that EGF and NGF may play a role in the ontogenesis of the human thymus as well as in the histogenesis of the thymomas. Hayashi and colleagues[47] reported an increasing level of expression of EGF and EGFR in increasingly malignant histology and in advanced stages versus early stages, and proposed a role for EGF and EGFR in thymoma progression. More recently, Ionescu and colleagues,[65] by means of an anti-EGFR mouse monoclonal antibody staining evaluated by the Dako score similarly to HER-2, found an EGFR protein overexpression in a high percentage of TET, which was not related to histotypes. Several articles[39,66,67] reported the overexpression of EGFR by IHC in advanced stages and in more malignant histotypes. EGFR overexpression was not related to mutational status (it appeared that EGFR mutations in TET are very rare)[67,68] and there was poor correlation between the EGFR protein expression and gene amplification[65] (only 7 of 23 specimens, 30% of cases) measured by fluorescent in situ hybridization (FISH) analysis using the dual-color EGFR SpectrumOrange/CEP7 SpectrumGreen probe Vysis. However, hyperploidy in invasive TET was also recorded. Meister and colleagues[68] first reported the use of the EGFR pharmDx kit Dako to evaluate EGFR staining. A high EGFR expression was found in the absence of statistically significant stage and histology correlation.

KIT as a Thymic Carcinoma Marker (and a Possible Target of Therapy?)

KIT (corresponding to CD117, a transmembrane tyrosine kinase receptor protein encoded by a proto-oncogene c-kit) is a molecule that triggers intracellular signals controlling cell proliferation and apoptosis. By performing an IHC on whole sections and TMA, KIT was found to be consistently expressed (heterogeneous or diffuse cytoplasmic staining) by thymic carcinomas but not by thymomas.[38] However, no mutations were found in the tumors (exons 9, 11 and exons 13 and 17). Similar data were provided by Henley and colleagues[39] and by Nagakawa and colleagues.[69] In the same year Stroebel and colleagues[70] described a c-kit activating mutation in thymic carcinomas in a tumor hyperexpressing KIT. The patient harboring the c-kit mutation was responsive for 6 months to imatinib therapy, then the disease progressed despite radiochemotherapy. A role for c-kit in TET oncogenesis was postulated. From further studies it appeared that KIT mutations, as well as EGFR mutations, are rare.[71]

ANGIOGENESIS MARKERS
Vascular Endothelial Growth Factors and Their Receptors (VEGFs and VEGFRs)

Angiogenesis is an essential and complex process necessary for the growth of all tumors, and therefore constitutes a potential target of therapy. The mammalian VEGF family consists of 5 glycoproteins referred to as VEGFA, VEGFB, VEGFC, VEGFD, and placental growth factor. The best characterized VEGFA, commonly referred to as VEGF, is the most powerful angiogenic factor known to date, and its levels are time-/space-correlated with phases of blood vessel growth. The VEGF ligands bind to and activate 3 structurally similar type III receptor tyrosine kinases (RTK), designated VEGFR1/FLT1, VEGFR2/KDR, and VEGFR3/FLT4. The assortment of VEGF ligands have distinctive binding specificities for each of these RTK, which contributes to their diversity of function. VEGFR2 expression is restricted primarily to the vasculature and is the key mediator of VEGF-induced angiogenesis. VEGFR1 is expressed on the vasculature as well but is also expressed on several other types of cells. VEGFR3 preferentially binds VEGFC and VEGFD; its expression in the adult is primarily on lymphatic endothelial cells, and it has a crucial role in postnatal lymphangiogenesis.[70] In addition to having proangiogenic effects, VEGF has several important functions that are independent of vascular processes, including autocrine effects on tumor cell function (survival, migration, invasion), immune suppression, and homing of bone marrow progenitors to prepare an organ for subsequent metastasis.[73]

Studies on angiogenic pathways in TET (46 cases from noninvasive thymoma to carcinoma) showed a significant correlation between tumor angiogenesis and invasiveness, and an association between VEGF expression and increased microvessel density.[74] Similar findings were reported by Kaira and colleagues.[25] Furthermore, Cimpean and colleagues[75] demonstrated the expression of VEGFR1, VEGFR2, and VEGFA in normal and pathologic conditions of thymus (including only 7 TETs) and suggested the possible use of antiangiogenic therapy. At present, a phase 2 study of erlotinib plus bevacizumab in advanced thymoma and thymic carcinomas is ongoing.[76]

Other Angiogenetic Markers: the COX-2 Protein

Considering the supposed protumorigenic potential of cyclooxygenase-2 (COX-2), an angiogenetic and apoptosis inhibitor, and the availability of COX-2 selective nonsteroidal anti-inflammatory drugs (NSAIDs) that can be considered anticancer drugs, COX-2 expression and up-regulation was studied in TET.[77] In normal thymuses COX-2 was found to be expressed only in medullary epithelial cells,[78] whereas in TET the expression of COX-2 was reported as moderate to strong. The 2 potential biomarkers, EGFR and COX-2, were significantly associated with the Spearman coefficient on studying 34 TET arrayed in TMA.[76] The eventual synergistic interaction of the EGFR and COX-2 pathways should be further investigated in TET.

PROGRESS IN METHODS TO APPROACH TET FOR BIOMARKER INVESTIGATIONS
TMA Technology

Biomarker studies in TET investigations hardly provide statistically significant data, as the rarity of these tumors prevents the collection of relevant case series. In addition, whole-section IHC significance is hampered by preanalytical differences in surgical procedures, sample handling conditions, tissue-embedding protocols, antibody batch applications, antigen retrieval methods, and incubation and washing times. In recent years, among the various high-throughput molecular technologies, TMA technology[79] has provided extensive knowledge on putative biomarkers that represent potential diagnostic, prognostic, and therapeutic targets in several tissues and tumors. The TMA is a validation and discovery platform that represents a translational research tool in biomarker profiling. The key benefit underlying TMA technology is its ability to assay up to hundreds of tissue samples arrayed on a single microscope slide. In its most usual form, a core of tissue is lifted from a formalin-fixed, paraffin-embedded sample and placed in a predrilled hole in a paraffin-recipient block. On sectioning, each sample is represented as a small (0.6–2 mm diameter) histologic section (histospot) arrayed in a grid that allows an easy link to clinicopathologic data. The result is a single slide that contains samples from 40 to 800 cases, depending on the core size. Due to the inherent efficiency in processing hundreds to thousands of tumors at one time, TMA dramatically increases the number of tumors that can be analyzed in a given cohort as compared with traditional whole-section studies. Larger cohorts positively affect the quality, significance, and reliability of the resulting biomarker studies. This fact is particularly true for biomarkers that are present in only a small percentage of tumors, in which smaller cohorts would provide insufficient numbers for statistical analysis. Given that TMA are arrayed on a single slide, all tumor specimens are stained consistently, at the same time, under the same conditions, and with exactly the same antibody dilution. Standardization and uniformity of the procedure is a marked difference from the traditional methods, in which batch-to-batch variability (and intervening time between batches) can have a profound effect on staining. TMA can easily be shared, providing a new outlet for performing multi-institutional studies using training and validation sets, which represent perhaps the best methods of assuring statistical value. TMA provide minimal tissue damage, cost reduction, and ease of interpretation, and save a significant amount of time.

TMA in TET

Previous studies
Very few examples of the use of TMA in TET are reported. The first example was in the KIT multitumor tissue microarray already mentioned.[38] Subsequently, the EGFR expression and distribution was investigated by Meister and colleagues[68] in a series of 20 TET, compared with the mutational analysis of the same cases as detected by direct sequencing of the EGFR gene. Therefore, the DNA-derived data were compared with the related protein expression. Dotto and colleagues[80] studied p63 distribution in 66 TET cases, which were evaluated by a semiquantitative assessment. A stronger expression of p63 was found in type B3

TET and in thymic carcinomas. The investigators suggested that this may be due to the amplification of the p63 gene.

TMA study of angiogenetic markers in TET

Recognition of the VEGF pathway as a key regulator of angiogenesis has led to the development of several VEGF-targeting agents that include neutralizing antibodies to VEGF or VEGFRs, soluble VEGF receptors or receptor hybrids, and TK inhibitors (TKIs) with selectivity for VEGFRs. So far, the anti-VEGF monoclonal antibody bevacizumab and the VEGFR TKIs sorafenib and sunitinib are currently approved by the US Food and Drug Administration for clinical use. It should be emphasized that owing to their mode of action at the adenosine triphosphate binding pocket, TKIs are selective rather than specific for a particular kinase(s). Thus, TKIs designed to target VEGF receptors are actually considered multi-kinase inhibitors. For example, sorafenib and sunitinib also have significant activity against platelet-derived growth factor receptor (PDGFR) and fibroblast growth factor receptor (FGFR), KIT, Raf, and FMS receptors.[81] Of note, some VEGFR-targeting TKIs significantly inhibit the activity of PDGFRs, whereby a dual attack on the vasculature (VEGFR on endothelial cells and PDGF on pericytes) in preclinical studies leads to greater efficacy than inhibiting a single receptor family.

From all these considerations and the studies previously reported, the authors investigated the expression of VEGF and their receptors, together with PDGFR, through the use of IHC in TET as potential therapeutic targets. The series included 100 TET (44 cases "low grade": A, AB, B1, MNT; and 56 cases "high grade": 32 cases B2, 16 cases B3, and 8 cases of carcinomas) collected in the framework of a multi-institutional collaborative project sponsored by the Italy-US Program (US and Italian National Institutes of Health) for Rare Diseases, arranged in TMA (**Fig. 3**). As reported in **Table 3**, distinct proportions of TET tumor cells expressed VEGFs and proangiogenic TK receptors. When compared with the low-grade counterpart, high-grade (B2, B3, carcinomas) TET were found to contain significantly higher numbers (t-test) of VEGFA, VEGFC, VEGFD, VEGFR1, and VEGFR2 expressing tumor cells (**Fig. 4**). Accordingly, increased circulating levels of VEGF were found in patients with thymic carcinoma but not thymomas.[82] In high-grade tumors, the smallest proportion of TKR immunoreactive cells were observed following staining for PDGFRβ. In addition, in high-grade TET, strong positive correlations between staining for VEGFA and those for all other markers were found (**Table 4**). In the same tumors, VEGFC staining was not associated with VEGFR1, VEGFR3, and PDGFRβ staining, and no correlation was obtained between VEGFD and VEGFR1 or VEGFR3 staining.

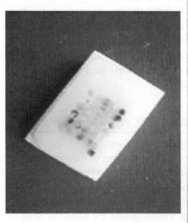
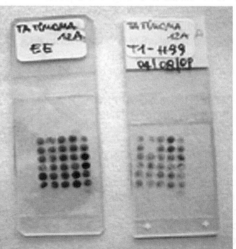

Fig. 3. Thymoma TMA. From left to right: paraffin block (2 mm cores), an H&E-stained slide, and a slide stained with anti-VEGFA primary antibody. The primary antibodies used in this study were: mouse monoclonal antibodies against VEGFA (Neomarkers, Fremont, CA), VEGFD (R&D Systems, Milan, Italy), and VEGFR3 (Monosan, Uden, The Netherlands); and polyclonal rabbit antibodies against VEGFC (Invitrogen, Camarillo, CA), VEGFR1 (Flt1) rabbit polyclonal (C-17) (Santa Cruz, Heidelberg, Germany), VEGFR2 (Flk1) rabbit polyclonal (C-1158) (Santa Cruz, Heidelberg, Germany), and PDGFRβ rabbit polyclonal (P-20) (Santa Cruz, Heidelberg, Germany). Secondary reagents were EnVision Mouse and EnVision Rabbit kits (DAKO, Milan, Italy).

Table 3
Angiogenetic marker expression in low-grade (A, AB, MNT, B1) and high-grade (B2, B3, carcinoma) TET

Marker	Low-Grade[a]	High-Grade[b]	P Value
VEGFA	39.6 ± 5.2[c]	55.8 ± 4.7	0.024[d]
VEGFC	29.2 ± 5.1	51.1 ± 4.7	0.003
VEGFD	27.2 ± 5.5	48.0 ± 4.6	0.005
VEGFR1	44.3 ± 6.9	65.5 ± 5.1	0.016
VEGFR2	50.1 ± 5.7	74.4 ± 3.6	0.001
VEGFR3	40.6 ± 5.4	52.8 ± 5.3	NS
PDGFRβ	17.4 ± 3.7	23.9 ± 4.0	NS

Abbreviations: NS, not significant; PDGFRβ, Platelet-derived growth factor receptor β; VEGFA, -C, -D, vascular endothelial growth factor A, C, and D; VEGFR1, -R2, -R3, vascular endothelial growth factor receptor 1, 2, and 3.
[a] n = 44.
[b] n = 56.
[c] Percent of positive tumor cells (mean ± SE).
[d] t-test.

In conclusion, TET expressed, in variable proportions, multiple potential targets of already available antiangiogenic treatments. However, to transform pharmacodynamic markers into predictive ones, clinical validation studies involving adequate numbers of patients are required.

Tissue-Based Targeted Therapies in TET

Targeted therapies are increasingly being applied experimentally in thymic tumors, even though the biologic basis of such therapies is not clearly defined. In 1997, based on the evidence of high

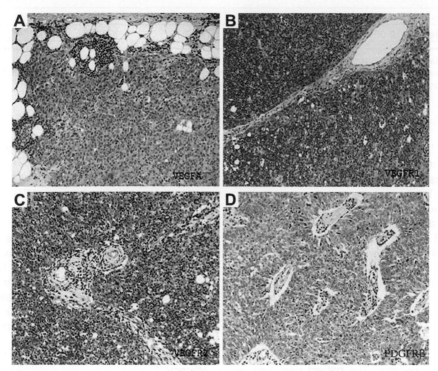

Fig. 4. Angiogenetic markers in TET TMA: in (*A*) stained with VEGFA (original magnification ×100), in (*B*) (×100) and C (×200) stained with VEGFR1 and VEGFR2, respectively; in (*D*) stained with antibody to PDGFRβ (×200). A moderate to strong cytoplasmic expression with each marker is presented. In (*A*) a type A thymoma, in (*B*) a type B2 thymoma, in (*C*) an AB thymoma, and in (*D*) a type B3 thymoma are shown. PDGFRβ, platelet-derived growth factor receptor β; VEGFA, vascular endothelial growth factor A; VEGFR1, -R2, vascular endothelial growth factor receptor 1 and 2, respectively.

Table 4
Spearman's correlation between markers in low-grade (A, AB, MNT, B1) and high-grade (B2, B3, carcinoma) TET

	VEGF-A	VEGF-C	VEGF-D	VEGFR1	VEGFR2	VEGFR3	PDGFRβ
VEGFA							
Low-grade[a]		NS	0.002	NS	0.025	NS	0.001
High-grade[b]		0.000[c]	0.005	0.003	0.000	0.013	0.001
VEGFC							
Low-grade	NS		0.000	NS	NS	NS	0.002
High-grade	0.000		0.000	NS	0.026	NS	NS
VEGFD							
Low-grade	0.002	0.000		NS	0.001	0.012	0.000
High-grade	0.005	0.000		NS	0.000	NS	0.005
VEGFR1							
Low-grade	NS	NS	NS		NS	NS	NS
High-grade	0.003	NS	NS		NS	NS	0.010
VEGFR2							
Low-grade	0.025	NS	0.001	NS		0.000	0.000
High-grade	0.000	0.026	0.000	NS		0.000	0.000
VEGFR3							
Low-grade	NS	NS	0.012	NS	0.000		0.022
High-grade	0.013	NS	NS	NS	0.000		0.000
PDGFRβ							
Low-grade	0.001	0.002	0.000	NS	0.000	0.022	
High-grade	0.001	NS	0.005	0.010	0.000	0.000	

Inverse correlations were not found.

Abbreviations: NS, not significant; PDGFRβ, platelet-derived growth factor receptor β; VEGFA, -C, -D, vascular endothelial growth factor A, C, and D; VEGFR1, -R2, -R3, vascular endothelial growth factor receptor 1, 2, and 3.

[a] n = 44.
[b] n = 56.
[c] *P* values for significant positive correlations.

uptake of [111]indium-labeled octreotide In-DTPA-D-Phe(1)-octreotide in thymic tumors, a patient was successfully treated with octreotide and prednisone.[83] The application of somatostatin analogues in this and in further cases was accredited to a high content of somatostatin receptors in TET.[84] The distribution of somatostatin receptors in the thymoma was subsequently described.[85,86] In the advanced stage of TET, a clinical trial later demonstrated a modest activity of the somatostatin analogues, which improved with prednisone association.[87,88] In more recent years, a patient suffering from imatinib-resistant BCR-ABL positive chronic myeloid leukemia in blast crisis was treated with dasatinib, a multitargeted kinase inhibitor. The patient was also reported to have had a reduction of a synchronous B2 stage I thymoma.[89] The thymoma showed low EGFR positivity, KIT negativity by IHC, and probable EGFR gene amplification by FISH analysis with the LSI EGFR/CEP7 probe. In 2007, 2 articles reported cetuximab responsiveness in 2 cases[90] and 1 case,[91] respectively. A tissue study was associated showing positive EGFR by IHC in both articles, and the absence of EGFR amplification detectable by FISH analysis in one of the articles.[91] In 2008, Christodoulou and colleagues[92] reported erlotinib responsiveness in an advanced TET. The TET treated showed positive EGFR by performing IHC; there was neither EGFR gene nor KIT gene mutation, nor EGFR amplification. Other cases of advanced thymic malignancies[93] were treated with the EGFR-tyrosine kinase inhibitor (EGFR-TKI), gefitinib. Recently, a phase 2 clinical trial with the combined use of TKI and an antiangiogenic drug was reported to have limited efficacy.[76]

New Perspectives

In rare tumors prognostic and predictive factors are very difficult to ascertain by a variety of approaches. Several pathways of oncological significance in TET were analyzed by different researchers performing IHC. However, it appears that both among "prognostic" markers and among pharmacogenomic/predictive markers, no definite answers were deemed to be clinically useful in TET patients. In fact the limited number of cases analyzed from each study certainly plays a role in rendering the ultimate goal so difficult to achieve. Modern medicine shows a trend toward an "early" detection of prognostic risk factors in each case. Predictive pathology in TET treatment is a young discipline. IHC has become a standard tool in diagnostic histopathology and in molecular pathology. IHC is also a powerful research tool in multimarker discovery study designs. This development is also associated with an increasing understanding of the complexity of tumor and normal tissue molecular biology and with the necessity to look at multiple factors for molecular phenotyping. Indeed, numerous types of post-translational modifications (ie, glycosylation, acylation, limited proteolysis, phosphorylation, isoprenylation) may modulate individual protein functions. Establishing functional cell lines from TET recently represented an important perspective tool in evaluating new therapeutic targets.[94] However, multicenter prospective studies based on a large series of cases will substantially enhance our knowledge of inherent biologic properties of single TET cases. Therefore, TMA appears to be a valuable tool for both biomarker validation in large TET case series and for the preliminary evaluation of the tumor in an individual patient enrolled in clinical trials.

SUMMARY

The role played by IHC in diagnostics and translational research in TET continues to be reviewed and discussed. As TET are rare tumors, the search for biomarkers of prognostic or predictive value is difficult. TMA technology appears to be a promising approach in TET. The authors' own data show the distribution and histotype correlation of VEGFs and VEGFRs in different TET groups derived from a TMA study and statistical analyses of 100 cases. TMA studies in rare tumors appear to provide a reproducible and statistically valid support in biomarker research, to be considered in multicenter studies for translational purposes and targeted therapy validation.

ACKNOWLEDGMENTS

The authors are grateful to Dr Rossano Lattanzio (Department of Oncology and Neurosciences, "G. D'Annunzio" University and Foundation Chieti-Pescara, Chieti, Italy) for his unvaluable collaboration, to Professor Francesco Facciolo (Thoracic Surgery, Regina Elena National Cancer Institute, Rome, Italy) for his continuous support, to Professor L. Lauriola (Department of Pathology, Catholic University of Rome, Italy) and to Professor Giovannella Palmieri (Department of Molecular and Clinical Endocrinology and Oncology, "Federico II" University, Naples, Italy) for the long-standing collaboration, and to R. Martucci for his excellent technical assistance. The authors would like to thank Professor Edoardo Pescarmona (Department of Pathology, Regina Elena National Cancer Institute, Rome, Italy) for helpful suggestions and Dr T. Merlino for English language editing.

REFERENCES

1. Travis WD. Pathology & genetics. Tumours of the lung, pleura, thymus and heart. Lyon (France): IARC Press; 2004.
2. Levine GD, Rosai J. Thymic hyperplasia and neoplasia: a review of current concepts. Hum Pathol 1978;9:495.
3. Marino M, Müller-Hermelink HK. Thymoma and thymic carcinoma. Relation of thymoma epithelial cells to the cortical and medullary differentiation of thymus. Virchows Arch A Pathol Anat Histopathol 1985;407:119.
4. Okumura M, Ohta M, Tateyama H, et al. The World Health Organization histologic classification system reflects the oncologic behavior of thymoma: a clinical study of 273 patients. Cancer 2002;94:624.
5. Chen G, Marx A, Wen-Hu C, et al. New WHO histologic classification predicts prognosis of thymic epithelial tumors: a clinicopathologic study of 200 thymoma cases from China. Cancer 2002;95:420.
6. Yamazaki K, Kitada M, Sasaki K, et al. [Surgery for thymomas and thymic carcinomas; treatment results in terms of WHO histologic typing, Masaoka staging system, and p53 expression]. Kyobu Geka 2002;55: 949 [in Japanese].
7. Rios A, Torres J, Galindo PJ, et al. Prognostic factors in thymic epithelial neoplasms. Eur J Cardiothorac Surg 2002;21:307.
8. Venuta F, Rendina EA, Longo F, et al. Long-term outcome after multimodality treatment for stage III thymic tumors. Ann Thorac Surg 2003;76:1866–72.
9. Park MS, Chung KY, Kim KD, et al. Prognosis of thymic epithelial tumors according to the new World Health Organization histologic classification. Ann Thorac Surg 2004;78:992.
10. Kondo K, Yoshizawa K, Tsuyuguchi M, et al. WHO histologic classification is a prognostic indicator in thymoma. Ann Thorac Surg 2004;77:1183.
11. Stroebel P, Bauer A, Puppe B, et al. Tumor recurrence and survival in patients treated for thymomas

and thymic squamous cell carcinomas: a retrospective analysis. J Clin Oncol 2004;22:1501.

12. Detterbeck FC. Clinical value of the WHO classification system of thymoma. Ann Thorac Surg 2006;81: 2328.

13. Kim DJ, Yang WI, Choi SS, et al. Prognostic and clinical relevance of the world health organization schema for the classification of thymic epithelial tumors: a clinicopathologic study of 108 patients and literature review. Chest 2005;127:755.

14. Honglin Y, Jun D, Zhenfeng L, et al. The correlation of the World Health Organization histologic classification of thymic epithelial tumors and its prognosis: a clinicopathologic study of 108 patients from China. Int J Surg Pathol 2009;17:255.

15. Okumura M, Shiono H, Minami M, et al. Clinical and pathological aspects of thymic epithelial tumors. Gen Thorac Cardiovasc Surg 2008;56:10.

16. Margaritora S, Cesario A, Cusumano G, et al. Thirty-five-year follow-up analysis of clinical and pathologic outcomes of thymoma surgery. Ann Thorac Surg 2010;89:245.

17. Venuta F, Anile M, Diso D, et al. Thymoma and thymic carcinoma. Eur J Cardiothorac Surg 2010; 37:13.

18. den Bakker MA, Oosterhuis JW. Tumours and tumour-like conditions of the thymus other than thymoma; a practical approach. Histopathology 2009; 54:69.

19. Suster S, Moran CA. Primary thymic epithelial neoplasms: spectrum of differentiation and histological features. Semin Diagn Pathol 1999;16:2.

20. Marchevsky AM, Gupta R, McKenna RJ, et al. Evidence-based pathology and the pathologic evaluation of thymomas: the World Health Organization classification can be simplified into only 3 categories other than thymic carcinoma. Cancer 2008;112: 2780.

21. Verghese ET, den Bakker MA, Campbell A, et al. Interobserver variation in the classification of thymic tumours—a multicentre study using the WHO classification system. Histopathology 2008;53:218.

22. Suster S, Moran CA. Thymoma, atypical thymoma, and thymic carcinoma. A novel conceptual approach to the classification of thymic epithelial neoplasms. Am J Clin Pathol 1999;111:826.

23. Nonaka D, Henley JD, Chiriboga L, et al. Diagnostic utility of thymic epithelial markers CD205 (DEC205) and Foxn1 in thymic epithelial neoplasms. Am J Surg Pathol 2007;31:1038.

24. Sarafian VS, Marinova TT, Gulubova MV. Differential expression of LAMPs and ubiquitin in human thymus. APMIS 2009;117:248.

25. Kaira K, Oriuchi N, Imai H, et al. L-type amino acid transporter 1 (LAT1) is frequently expressed in thymic carcinomas but is absent in thymomas. J Surg Oncol 2009;99:433.

26. Raica M, Kondylis A, Mogoanta L, et al. Diagnostic and clinical significance of D2-40 expression in the normal human thymus and thymoma. Rom J Morphol Embryol 2010;51:229.

27. Pomplun S, Wotherspoon AC, Shah G, et al. Immunohistochemical markers in the differentiation of thymic and pulmonary neoplasms. Histopathology 2002;40:152.

28. Attanoos RL, Galateau-Salle F, Gibbs AR, et al. Primary thymic epithelial tumours of the pleura mimicking malignant mesothelioma. Histopathology 2002;41:42.

29. Pan CC, Chen PC, Chou TY, et al. Expression of calretinin and other mesothelioma-related markers in thymic carcinoma and thymoma. Hum Pathol 2003;34:1155.

30. Mueller-Hermelink HK, Marino M, Palestro G, et al. Immunohistological evidences of cortical and medullary differentiation in thymoma. Virchows Arch A Pathol Anat Histopathol 1985;408:143.

31. Kodama T, Watanabe S, Sato Y, et al. An immunohistochemical study of thymic epithelial tumors. I. Epithelial component. Am J Surg Pathol 1986;10:26.

32. Kuo T. Cytokeratin profiles of the thymus and thymomas: histogenetic correlations and proposal for a histological classification of thymomas. Histopathology 2000;36:403.

33. Chilosi M, Castelli P, Martignoni G, et al. Neoplastic epithelial cells in a subset of human thymomas express the B cell-associated CD20 antigen. Am J Surg Pathol 1992;16:988.

34. Hishima T, Fukayama M, Fujisawa M, et al. CD5 expression in thymic carcinoma. Am J Pathol 1994; 145:268.

35. Dorfman DM, Shahsafaei A, Chan JK. Thymic carcinomas, but not thymomas and carcinomas of other sites, show CD5 immunoreactivity. Am J Surg Pathol 1997;21:936.

36. Kornstein MJ, Rosai J. CD5 labeling of thymic carcinomas and other nonlymphoid neoplasms. Am J Clin Pathol 1998;109:722.

37. Tateyama H, Eimoto T, Tada T, et al. Immunoreactivity of a new CD5 antibody with normal epithelium and malignant tumors including thymic carcinoma. Am J Clin Pathol 1999;111:235.

38. Pan CC, Chen PC, Chiang H. KIT (CD117) is frequently overexpressed in thymic carcinomas but is absent in thymomas. J Pathol 2004;202:375.

39. Henley JD, Cummings OW, Loehrer PJ, et al. Tyrosine kinase receptor expression in thymomas. J Cancer Res Clin Oncol 2004;130:222.

40. Kirchner T, Schalke B, Buchwald J, et al. Well-differentiated thymic carcinoma. An organotypical low-grade carcinoma with relationship to cortical thymoma. Am J Surg Pathol 1992;16:1153.

41. Kuo TT, Chang JP, Lin FJ, et al. Thymic carcinomas: histopathological varieties and immunohistochemical study. Am J Surg Pathol 1990;14:24.

42. Suster S, Rosai J. Thymic carcinoma. A clinicopathologic study of 60 cases. Cancer 1991;67:1025.

43. Suster S, Moran CA. Spindle cell thymic carcinoma: clinicopathologic and immunohistochemical study of a distinctive variant of primary thymic epithelial neoplasm. Am J Surg Pathol 1999;23:691.

44. Stroebel P, Marino M, Feuchtenberger M, et al. Micronodular thymoma: an epithelial tumour with abnormal chemokine expression setting the stage for lymphoma development. J Pathol 2005;207:72.

45. Yoneda S, Marx A, Mueller-Hermelink HK. Low-grade metaplastic carcinomas of the thymus: biphasic thymic epithelial tumors with mesenchymal metaplasia—an update. Pathol Res Pract 1999;195:555.

46. Brown JG, Familiari U, Papotti M, et al. Thymic basaloid carcinoma: a clinicopathologic study of 12 cases, with a general discussion of basaloid carcinoma and its relationship with adenoid cystic carcinoma. Am J Surg Pathol 2009;33:1113.

47. Hayashi Y, Ishii N, Obayashi C, et al. Thymoma: tumour type related to expression of epidermal growth factor (EGF), EGF-receptor, p53, v-erb B and ras p21. Virchows Arch 1995;426:43.

48. Tateyama H, Eimoto T, Tada T, et al. p53 protein expression and p53 gene mutation in thymic epithelial tumors. An immunohistochemical and DNA sequencing study. Am J Clin Pathol 1995;104:375.

49. Hirabayashi H, Fujii Y, Sakaguchi M, et al. p16INK4, pRB, p53 and cyclin D1 expression and hypermethylation of CDKN2 gene in thymoma and thymic carcinoma. Int J Cancer 1997;73:639.

50. Hino N, Kondo K, Miyoshi T, et al. High frequency of p53 protein expression in thymic carcinoma but not in thymoma. Br J Cancer 1997;76:1361.

51. Weirich G, Schneider P, Fellbaum C, et al. p53 alterations in thymic epithelial tumours. Virchows Arch 1997;431:17.

52. Hiroshima K, Iyoda A, Toyozaki T, et al. Proliferative activity and apoptosis in thymic epithelial neoplasms. Mod Pathol 2002;15:1326.

53. Baldi A, Ambrogi V, Mineo D, et al. Analysis of cell cycle regulator proteins in encapsulated thymomas. Clin Cancer Res 2005;11:5078.

54. Mineo TC, Ambrogi V, Baldi A, et al. Recurrent intrathoracic thymomas: potential prognostic importance of cell-cycle protein expression. J Thorac Cardiovasc Surg 2009;138:40.

55. Mineo TC, Ambrogi V, Mineo D, et al. Long-term disease-free survival of patients with radically resected thymomas: relevance of cell-cycle protein expression. Cancer 2005;104:2063.

56. Khoury T, Arshad A, Bogner P, et al. Apoptosis-related (survivin, Bcl-2), tumor suppressor gene (p53), proliferation (Ki-67), and nonreceptor tyrosine kinase (Src) markers expression and correlation with clinicopathologic variables in 60 thymic neoplasms. Chest 2009;136:220.

57. Di Como CJ, Urist MJ, Babayan I, et al. p63 expression profiles in human normal and tumor tissues. Clin Cancer Res 2002;8:494.

58. Chilosi M, Zamò A, Brighenti A, et al. Constitutive expression of DeltaN-p63alpha isoform in human thymus and thymic epithelial tumours. Virchows Arch 2003;443:175.

59. Kikuchi T, Ichimiya S, Kojima T, et al. Expression profiles and functional implications of p53-like transcription factors in thymic epithelial cell subtypes. Int Immunol 2004;16:831.

60. Wu M, Sun K, Gil J, et al. Immunohistochemical detection of p63 and XIAP in thymic hyperplasia and thymomas. Am J Clin Pathol 2009;131:689.

61. Chen FF, Yan JJ, Chang KC, et al. Immunohistochemical localization of Mcl-1 and bcl-2 proteins in thymic epithelial tumours. Histopathology 1996;29:541.

62. Pan CC, Chen PC, Wang LS, et al. Expression of apoptosis-related markers and HER-2/neu in thymic epithelial tumours. Histopathology 2003;43:165.

63. Salakou S, Tsamandas AC, Bonikos DS, et al. The potential role of bcl-2, bax, and Ki67 expression in thymus of patients with myasthenia gravis, and their correlation with clinicopathologic parameters. Eur J Cardiothorac Surg 2001;20:712.

64. Pescarmona E, Pisacane A, Pignatelli E, et al. Expression of epidermal and nerve growth factor receptors in human thymus and thymomas. Histopathology 1993;23:39.

65. Ionescu DN, Sasatomi E, Cieply K, et al. Protein expression and gene amplification of epidermal growth factor receptor in thymomas. Cancer 2005;103:630.

66. Gilhus NE, Jones M, Turley H, et al. Oncogene proteins and proliferation antigens in thymomas: increased expression of epidermal growth factor receptor and Ki67 antigen. J Clin Pathol 1995;48:447.

67. Suzuki E, Sasaki H, Kawano O, et al. Expression and mutation statuses of epidermal growth factor receptor in thymic epithelial tumors. Jpn J Clin Oncol 2006;36:351.

68. Meister M, Schirmacher P, Dienemann H, et al. Mutational status of the epidermal growth factor receptor (EGFR) gene in thymomas and thymic carcinomas. Cancer Lett 2007;248:186.

69. Nakagawa K, Matsuno Y, Kunitoh H, et al. Immunohistochemical KIT (CD117) expression in thymic epithelial tumors. Chest 2005;128:140.

70. Stroebel P, Hartmann M, Jakob A, et al. Thymic carcinoma with overexpression of mutated KIT and the response to imatinib. N Engl J Med 2004;350:2625.

71. Yoh K, Nishiwaki Y, Ishii G, et al. Mutational status of EGFR and KIT in thymoma and thymic carcinoma. Lung Cancer 2008;62:316.

72. Ellis LM, Hicklin DJ. VEGF-targeted therapy: mechanisms of anti-tumour activity. Nat Rev Cancer 2008; 8:579.

73. Kaplan RN, Riba RD, Zacharoulis S, et al. VEGFR1-positive haematopoietic bone marrow progenitors initiate the pre-metastatic niche. Nature 2005;438:820.

74. Tomita M, Matsuzaki Y, Edagawa M, et al. Correlation between tumor angiogenesis and invasiveness in thymic epithelial tumors. J Thorac Cardiovasc Surg 2002;124:493.

75. Cimpean AM, Raica M, Encica S, et al. Immunohistochemical expression of vascular endothelial growth factor A (VEGF), and its receptors (VEGFR1, 2) in normal and pathologic conditions of the human thymus. Ann Anat 2008;190:238.

76. Bedano PM, Perkins S, Burns M, et al. A phase II trial of erlotinib plus bevacizumab in patients with recurrent thymoma or thymic carcinoma [abstract 19087]. ASCO Annual Meeting Proceedings. J Clin Oncol 2008;26.

77. Rieker RJ, Joos S, Mechtersheimer G, et al. COX-2 upregulation in thymomas and thymic carcinomas. Int J Cancer 2006;119:2063.

78. Rocca B, Maggiano N, Habib A, et al. Distinct expression of cyclooxygenase-1 and -2 in the human thymus. Eur J Immunol 2002;32:1482.

79. Kallioniemi OP, Wagner U, Kononen J, et al. Tissue microarray technology for high-throughput molecular profiling of cancer. Hum Mol Genet 2001;10:657.

80. Dotto J, Pelosi G, Rosai J. Expression of p63 in thymomas and normal thymus. Am J Clin Pathol 2007; 127:415.

81. Karaman MW, Herrgard S, Treiber DK, et al. A quantitative analysis of kinase inhibitor selectivity. Nat Biotechnol 2008;26:127.

82. Sasaki H, Yukiue H, Kobayashi Y, et al. Elevated serum vascular endothelial growth factor and basic fibroblast growth factor levels in patients with thymic epithelial neoplasms. Surg Today 2001;31:1038.

83. Palmieri G, Lastoria S, Colao A, et al. Successful treatment of a patient with a thymoma and pure red-cell aplasia with octreotide and prednisone. N Engl J Med 1997;336:263.

84. Palmieri G, Montella L, Martignetti A, et al. Somatostatin analogs and prednisone in advanced refractory thymic tumors. Cancer 2002;94:1414.

85. Ferone D, Kwekkeboom DJ, Pivonello R, et al. In vivo and in vitro expression of somatostatin receptors in two human thymomas with similar clinical presentation and different histological features. J Endocrinol Invest 2001;24:522.

86. Ferone D, Montella L, De Chiara A, et al. Somatostatin receptor expression in thymic tumors. Front Biosci 2009;14:3304.

87. Loehrer PJ Sr, Wang W, Johnson DH, et al. Octreotide alone or with prednisone in patients with advanced thymoma and thymic carcinoma: an Eastern Cooperative Oncology Group Phase II trial. J Clin Oncol 2004;22:293.

88. Kurup A, Loehrer PJ Sr. Thymoma and thymic carcinoma: therapeutic approaches. Clin Lung Cancer 2004;6:28.

89. Chuah C, Lim TH, Lim AS, et al. Dasatinib induces a response in malignant thymoma. J Clin Oncol 2006;24:e56.

90. Palmieri G, Marino M, Salvatore M, et al. Cetuximab is an active treatment of metastatic and chemorefractory thymoma. Front Biosci 2007;12:757.

91. Farina G, Garassino MC, Gambacorta M, et al. Response of thymoma to cetuximab. Lancet Oncol 2007;8:449.

92. Christodoulou C, Murray S, Dahabreh J, et al. Response of malignant thymoma to erlotinib. Ann Oncol 2008;19(7):1361–2.

93. Kurup A. Phase II study of gefitinib treatment in advanced thymic malignancies. J Clin Oncol 2005; 23:16s.

94. Ehemann V, Kern MA, Breinig M, et al. Establishment, characterization and drug sensitivity testing in primary cultures of human thymoma and thymic carcinoma. Int J Cancer 2008;122: 2719.

Management of Myasthenic Patients with Thymoma

Marcin Zieliński, MD, PhD

KEYWORDS

- Thymus • Mediastinum • Myasthenia gravis
- Thymoma • Surgery

Thymomas are primary neoplasms of the thymus gland originating from the thymic epithelial cells that present no cytologic or histologic signs of malignancy. The other thymic tumors such as lymphomas, dysgerminal tumors, or carcinoids are not thymomas. A well-differentiated thymic carcinoma presents some cytologic features of atypia, and thymic cancer cells are cytologically malignant.[1–3] Thymic carcinoma comprises less than 10% of all thymomas, is rarely accompanied by myasthenia gravis (MG), is usually symptomatic, and has worse prognosis than other thymomas.[4,5] Thymomas are the most prevalent tumors of the anterior mediastinum, comprising about 50% of tumors of the anterior mediastinum and 15% to 20% of all mediastinal tumors. About 15% of all patients with MG have thymomas, and 35% patients with thymomas have MG.[5,6] Pathomechanism of MG associated with thymoma is complex and understood only in part. Probably, the mechanisms of MG in thymomas and nonthymomatous MG are different. Complete description of the mechanisms of development of MG associated with thymomas is beyond the scope of this article.[7]

This review analyzes some issues of surgical treatment of patients with thymoma-associated MG.

A search of the MEDLINE database was performed with the keywords thymoma, myasthenia gravis, recurrence of thymoma, and surgery. Only English-language articles published after 1990 were included. Selected, important, frequently cited articles published before this date were also included. The inclusion criteria for surgical series were at least 50 patients operated on for thymoma and all publications on minimally invasive techniques of thymectomy for thymomas, on surgery of MG-associated thymomas, and on reoperation for recurrence. In case of several articles by the same investigators, the recently updated publications were chosen.

The exclusion criteria were case series, surgery for nonthymomatous MG, and articles on surgery, chemotherapy, chemoradiotherapy, and radiotherapy for non-MG thymomas.

CHARACTERISTICS OF THYMOMA ASSOCIATED WITH MG

Thymomas are relatively rare tumors—the annual incidence in the United States is 0.15 new cases per 100,000 population.[8] Thymomas occur more frequently in patients of Chinese origin (48%) with MG than those of White race. Patients of Chinese origin with MG had fewer severe cases and significantly lower anti–acetylcholine receptor (anti-AChR) antibody titers than patients of White race. The racial heterogeneity of MG suggests that thymomas occur in genetically predisposed individuals.[9–11] Mean age of patients with thymoma-associated MG was 49.2 ± 13.3,[12] 47.26 ± 14.44, 47.66,[13] 44.9,[14] and 44.0 years,[15] without significant differences between male/female rate. Patients with thymoma-associated MG tend to be significantly younger than those with non-MG thymoma.[12] Mean duration of MG from the onset of symptoms to thymectomy was 1.06 ± 3.38 years,[16] with 92.5% of patients undergoing thymectomy within 3 years from the onset of

Department of Thoracic Surgery, Pulmonary Hospital, Ul. Gładkie 1, 34 500 Zakopane, Poland
E-mail address: marcinz@mp.pl

Thorac Surg Clin 21 (2011) 47–57
doi:10.1016/j.thorsurg.2010.08.009
1547-4127/11/$ — see front matter © 2011 Elsevier Inc. All rights reserved.

MG which was significantly shorter than that of nonthymomatous MG.[15] Several large series of thymomas with associated MG included 3% Osserman grade I, 34.5% grade IIA, 53% grade IIB, and 9.2% grade III[14,17] and Myasthenia Gravis Foundation of America (MGFA) classification grade I 1.93%, grade II 27.1%, grade III 37.7%, and grade IV 10.6%.[13,18] According to World Health Organization (WHO) classification, the incidence of MG in thymomas was the highest in the subtypes B2, B1, and AB and the incidence in subtypes A and B3 was 10% or less (**Table 1**).[13,16,19–21]

The distribution of the histologic types of thymoma was similar in the groups with and without associated MG.[12] Antititin and antiryanodine receptor antibodies are found in up to 95% of patients with MG with thymoma; therefore, their detection can be valuable in diagnostics.[22,23]

SURGICAL TREATMENT OF THYMOMAS

There is a general agreement that Masaoka stage I and WHO types A and AB thymomas should undergo primary resection without any adjuvant therapy, with survival prognosis on recurrence reaching almost 100%.[5,24] The role of adjuvant radiotherapy or chemoradiotherapy after thymectomy has been questioned for stage II and stage III thymomas, especially for WHO B1 to B3 types.[24–26] The policy of neoadjuvant and adjuvant therapy is the same for thymomas associated or not associated with MG and is not analyzed in this article. There are several types of operative approaches for the removal of thymomas. The traditional approach through of complete median sternotomy is still regarded as the gold standard for treating thymomas. This approach is used by most thoracic surgeons, especially for Masaoka stage II to III thymomas.[5,6,15] This approach is regarded to be the safest in avoidance of injury of the tumor capsule, which is presumably the factor that might lead to the local recurrence. There are 3 types of surgical procedures for thymomas with regard to the extensiveness of removal of the thymus gland and the surrounding tissue: (1) resection of the tumor and a part of the thymus, leaving the rest of the thymus behind, (2) thymothymectomy or thymomectomy (resection of the whole thymus containing thymoma), and (3) extended thymectomy (resection of the whole thymus and the surrounding adipose tissue of the neck and the mediastinum).[12] The reasons to perform thymothymectomy (thymomectomy) include elimination of possible multicentric growth of the thymoma in the thymus and minimization of the risk of occurrence of MG after thymectomy.[27,28] Regnard and colleagues[28] found a second thymoma in 8 of 307 operations.

The possible justification for the use of extended thymectomy is to remove the ectopic foci of the thymic tissue.[14,18] This approach has been supported with occasional discovery of ectopic thymomas developing from the main thymus gland.[29–31] The other reason to perform extended thymectomy is the possible influence on the development of MG because of the presence of the retained ectopic thymic foci. However, there has been no evidence supporting this approach.

MINIMALLY INVASIVE TECHNIQUES OF THYMECTOMY FOR THYMOMAS

During the last 2 decades, minimally invasive techniques of thymectomy for MG have been

Table 1
Incidence of MG in different types of thymomas according to the WHO histologic classification of thymomas

Authors	No. of Patients	Type A (%)	Type AB (%)	Type B1 (%)	Type B2 (%)	Type B3 (%)	Type C (%)	Other Types (%)
Evoli et al,[13] 2002	207	2.1	10.1	22.3	55.3	3.2	—	6.4
Maggi et al,[16] 2008	197	10.7	28.4	14.7	31.0	9.6	—	3.6
Margaritora et al,[19] 2010	276	ns	ns	ns	ns	ns	ns	a
Chen et al,[20] 2002	30	25	7.8	17.6	38.2	29.6	2.7	—
Okumura et al,[21] 2002	127	16.7	15.6	56.4	71.1	46.2	46.2	0

Abbreviation: ns, not stated.
a MG was associated significantly more frequently with types B1 and B2 than with the other subtypes (*P*<.001).

developed, mainly for the treatment of nonthymomatous MG. The minimally invasive techniques are those that use operative approaches without sternotomy. These techniques include transcervical, videothoracoscopic (VATS), and subxiphoid approaches or a combination of these approaches. The advantages of minimally invasive techniques include less pain in the early postoperative period, less-compromised pulmonary function, better cosmetic result, and total avoidance of the risk of disruption or infection of the sternotomy wound.[32,33] Disadvantages of VATS approach include insufficient completeness of removal of the upper poles of the thymus[33] with unilateral or bilateral VATS approach, risk of chronic pain after thoracoscopy in 10% of patients,[34] and an unproven oncological usefulness in thymomas, with only 1 report including more than 50 patients with thymoma and follow-up of at least 5 years. Several surgical teams started to use less-invasive approaches, including the transcervical incision with elevation of the sternal manubrium with mechanical retractor, unilateral left-sided and right-sided VATS approach,[35–37] bilateral VATS approach,[38] combined approach,[39–41] transcervical approach,[42,43] or infrasternal approach for the treatment of the early-stage thymomas (see **Table 1**).[42–49]

Odaka and colleagues[44] used unilateral thoracoscopic subtotal thymectomy for stage I and stage II thymomas. The preliminary results of this study suggested that thoracoscopic thymectomy was feasible, safe, and less invasive in comparison to the transsternal technique. No recurrence of thymoma was noted in the thoracoscopic group during a median follow-up period of 21.6 months (range, 5–40 months). Maggi and colleagues[16] analyzed thymoma-associated MG in a group of patients operated on with transsternal and video-assisted thoracoscopic extended thymectomy (VATET) approaches, with a mean follow-up of 7.69 ± 6.0 years. The whole group included 197 patients, and the VATET subgroup included 71 patients. The investigators found no differences in the complete remission rates and recurrence rates between trassternal and VATET subgroups; however, the complete remission rate was only 9.64% for thymoma-associated MG. Until now, this is the only reported series of minimally invasive thymectomy for MG associated with thymomas, including more than 50 patients with a mean follow-up exceeding 5 years. Cheng and colleagues[45] found no difference in survival in the mean follow-up period of 33.9 ± 19.7 months between 12 patients who underwent VATS procedure and 10 patients who underwent trassternal thymectomy for stage II thymomas. Soon and

Agasthian[46] reported the use of VATS thymectomy in 49 patients with thymoma. The investigators found the use of harmonic scalpel to be safe and advantageous when compared with the conventional technique of monopolar electrocautery and Vascular Clips however, the duration of follow-up was relatively short, 3.40 ± 2.38 years (range, 0.04–8.52 years).[47] Thoracoscopic thymectomy can be performed with the use of da Vinci robotic system. Augustin and colleagues[50] operated on 9 patients with thymoma and Savitt and colleagues[51] on 14 patients with thymoma, including 1 patient who underwent biopsy of the tumor and 3 patients who switched to treatment with sternotomy because of the extracapsular invasion of the tumor. The largest series of 30 robotic thymectomies for thymomas was presented by Rückert and colleagues.[52] Most thoracic surgeons agree that such procedures should be limited to small thymomas that are easily removable from the chest with low risk of injury to the capsule. A maximum diameter of 4 cm has been proposed for such less-invasive techniques[38] however, Odaka and colleagues[44] removed thymomas of the diameter 44 ± 18.9 mm, and Soon and Agasthian[46] removed thymomas of the diameter 40 ± 20.8 mm and 56.6 ± 18.2 mm, with or without the use of harmonic scalpel, respectively. Shigemura and colleagues[33] found that thoracoscopic thymectomy often results in retaining parts of the upper poles of the thymus in the neck. However, contrary to nonthymomatous MG, subtotal thymectomy might not be critically important if the whole tumor is completely resected. Transcervical approach for thymectomy for MG associated with thymoma was used extensively by Papatestas and colleagues[42] who performed 64 operations for Masaoka stages I, II, and III thymomas using this technique, including 11 tumors greater than 5 cm diameter, without any postoperative mortality. Subsequently, transcervical thymectomy for thymoma was abandoned for more than 1 decade. The use of transcervical thymectomy for thymoma was reported by Deeb and colleagues,[43] who performed 14 procedures with shifts to sternotomy or VATS in 5 of 14 patients.

Infrasternal approach for thymectomy of thymomas associated with MG was used in 16 patients by Uchiyama and colleagues,[48] with 2 patients with Masaoka stage III thymomas necessitating a change to sternotomy. Sakamaki and colleagues[49] reported results of 30 patients with noninvasive thymomas. Unilateral thoracoscopic partial (or subtotal) thymectomy (UTPT) was performed on 11 nonmyasthenic patients, and infrasternal mediastinal thymectomy (ETIS) was performed on 19 patients (13 myasthenic and 6 nonmyasthenic patients). In the ETIS group, 3 patients underwent a change to sternotomy because of pericardial dissemination, pleural adhesion, and vascular injury, respectively. The mean surgical duration was 163 and 224 minutes and mean blood loss was 123 and 149 g for UTPT and ETIS, respectively. Postthymomectomy MG occurred after UTPT in a patient who made an excellent recovery to remission after the re-UTPT. No recurrence was detected for 48 months of mean postoperative follow-up.

Analyzing the results of these up to now largest series of minimally invasive thymectomies, it must be stressed that the mean time interval from thymectomy to local recurrence of thymoma is more than 7 years; hence, it is too early to estimate the real oncological value of these approaches.

PREOPERATIVE AND POSTOPERATIVE TREATMENT OF PATIENTS WITH THYMOMA ASSOCIATED WITH MG

A substantial number of patients with MG associated with thymoma need administration of immunosuppressive drugs (including corticosteroids), plasmapheresis, intravenous immunoglobulins (IVIG), or other drugs (tacrolimus, mycophenolate mofetil).[13,53] The preoperative use of immunosuppressive drugs is highly variable and ranges from 4.1%[15] to 100%.[54] López-Cano and colleagues[55] used steroids preoperatively in 66.7% of patients, and Maggi and colleagues[16] administered steroids, immunosuppressive drugs, and both in 81.7%, 3.1%, and 60.9% of patients, respectively. In addition, plasmapheresis and IVIG were administered at least once in 44.7% patients. Maggi and colleagues[14] administered steroids and plasmapheresis in 25.7% and 6.8% of patients, respectively (there was no difference with the rate of use of these modalities in comparison to the patients with nonthymomatous MG). Evoli and colleagues[13] reported that 59.6% of patients were taking immunosuppressive drugs preoperatively. Generally, more patients with thymoma associated with MG needed immunosuppressive drugs preoperatively in comparison to the reported data regarding patients with nonthymomatous MG. The postoperative rate of use of immunosuppressive drugs and plasmapheresis was higher than the preoperative period in patients with MG associated with thymoma. About 81.6% of patients reported by Evoli and colleagues[13] received immunosuppressive treatment during follow-up, and Maggi and colleagues[16] administered steroids, azathioprine,

and plasmapheresis in 68%, 40.7%, and 21.6% of patients, respectively.

About 22.7% of patients experienced one or more respiratory crises during the course of the disease,[13] whereas according to the study by Maggi and colleagues,[16] it was 21.3%. Respiratory failure rates after thymectomy ranged from 2.2%[19] to 29.6%[28] and 40.7%.[55]

OUTCOME OF PATIENTS WITH THYMOMA ASSOCIATED WITH MG

Long-term survival rates after resection of thymomas are related to the histologic type of thymoma according to the Muller-Hermelink and WHO classifications and the Masaoka stages. Almost 100% recurrence-free survival rates were reported in type A (medullary thymomas) in the Masaoka stage I. On the other hand, in stage III thymic cancer (type C), 5-year survival rates of 20% to 40% were reported. The results of the series including more than 100 patients with thymoma associated with MG showed consistently that prognosis for long-term survival is better in case of thymomas associated with MG than non-MG thymomas (**Table 2**).

OUTCOME OF PATIENTS WITH MG ASSOCIATED WITH THYMOMA

The results of treatment of MG associated with thymomas reported in the largest series including more than 100 patients are generally worse than those in patients with nonthymomatous MG (**Table 3**). According to most of the investigators, complete remission rates usually do not exceed 10% to 20% after 5 years' follow-up of thymectomy in MG-associated thymomas when compared with 30% to 60% in nonthymomatous MG (**Table 4**).[12–16,42] However, such differences have not been shown in several studies including less that 100 patients and therefore not analyzed in this article.

MG OCCURRING AFTER RESECTION OF THYMOMA

MG associated with thymoma is often exacerbated after removal of thymoma. Somnier[9] found that the myasthenic symptoms were aggravated in most patients after thymectomy for thymoma, which was accompanied by increase in anti-AChR antibody titers. The peak of this process was achieved approximately after 300 days of thymectomy and lasted up to 3 years. About 20.6% of patients experienced deterioration of MG in the first year after thymectomy.[13] Exacerbation of MG after removal of thymoma has also

Table 2
Minimally invasive thymectomy series, including more than 10 patients

Authors	Technique of Thymectomy	No. of Patients/ No. of Patients with MG	Masaoka Stage	Follow-up	Effect on MG (% of CR)	No. of Recurrences (%)
Papatestas et al,[42] 1987	Transcervical basic	64	I–III	ns	ns	ns
Roviaro et al,[38] 2000	Bilateral VATS	22/ns	I	ns	ns	ns
Deeb et al,[43] 2001	Transcervical	14/14	I-5 II-8 III-1	Mean 48 mo (3–96 mo)	ns	0
Uchiyama et al,[48] 2004	Substernal VATS	16/11	I-13 II-1 III-2	Mean 19.2 mo (2–33 mo)	11.1	0
Cheng et al,[46] 2005	Unilateral VATS subtotal, 12; transsternal, 10	22/ns	II	33.9 ± 19.7 mo	ns	0, no difference of survival
Sakamaki et al,[49] 2008	Unilateral VATS subtotal, 11; infrasternal mediastinal total, 19	30/13	ns	48	ns	0
Maggi et al,[16] 2008	VATET, 71; extended transsternal, 126	197/197	I–IV	Mean 7.69 ± 6.0 y	9.64	9.64 (no difference between VATET and transsternal)
Agasthian Lin,[47] 2010	Unilateral VATS subtotal	58/32	I–IVA	Mean 4.9 y (1.9–10 y)	21	3.44
Odaka et al,[44] 2010	Unilateral VATS subtotal	22/0	I–II	Mean 21.6 mo (5–40 mo)	—	0
Rückert et al,[52] 2010	Unilateral VATS robotic, 30; transsternal, 44	74/ns	ns	ns	No difference in CR	No difference in survival

Abbreviations: CR, complete remission; ns, not stated.

Table 3
Influence of MG on survival in thymomas in the series including more than 100 patients

Authors	No. of Patients with Thymoma/No. of Patients with Thymoma Associated with MG	Follow-up	Effect of MG on Survival
Margaritora et al,[19] 2010	317/276	144.7 ± 104.4 mo	5- and 10-y survival was 90% and 86% for thymomas associated with MG and 85% and 75% for thymomas without MG, respectively; $P = .046$
Kondo and Monden,[12] 2005	1089/270	5 y	Trend for better 5-y survival for stage IV thymomas associated with MG is 89.3% vs 63.9% for thymomas without MG; $P = .0523$ Resectability is higher for thymomas associated with MG than for thymomas without MG, 60% vs 38%
Maggi et al,[14] 1991	241/160	ns	5- and 10-y survival is 85% and 82% for thymomas associated with MG and 78% and 67% for thymomas without MG, respectively
Okumura et al,[68] 1999	194/109	11.3 ± 7.8 y	Trend for better 10- and 20-y survival is 91% and 73% for thymomas associated with MG vs 82% and 69% for thymomas without MG, respectively; $P = .07$
Regnard et al,[28] 1996	307/197	Median 5.5 y (1–28 y)	10-y survival is 70% for thymomas associated with MG and 62% for thymomas without MG, respectively; $P > .05$
Okumura et al,[21] 2002	273/127	Mean 11.3 ± 7.8 y	MG has no effect on survival in multivariate analysis; $P = .48$

been reported.[56,57] In patients with non-MG thymoma, MG occurs after thymectomy. This occurrence might indicate a recurrence of thymoma, but MG can also occur without a recurrence of thymoma.

The risk of occurrence of MG after removal of thymoma without associated MG is 1% to 3%.[58,59] Nakajima and colleagues[60] found that patients in whom postthymectomy MG developed showed high titers of AChR-binding antibodies at the onset of MG. The investigators concluded that positive preoperative AChR antibody levels may be a risk factor for postthymectomy MG. Similar observations have been made by Toong and colleagues.[61] The interval between a

thymectomy and the onset of postoperative MG is variable (6 days–45 months; mean, 19 months).[27] There was no relation between the appearance of postoperative MG and histologic type of thymoma and the type of surgical procedure (resection of the tumor, thymothymectomy, extended thymectomy). Postoperative MG included pure ocular or generalized disease, which was responsive to medical treatment with anticholinesterase and/or steroids.[27] Maggi and colleagues[16] reported the occurrence of MG after thymectomy for thymoma in 9.6% of patients. MG developed during the first 2 years after surgery in all but 1 patient. In 89.5% (17 of 19) of patients, there was an invasive thymoma, and only 1 patient

Table 4
Complete remission rate of thymoma associated with MG in the series including more than 100 patients

Authors	No. of Patients with MG-Associated Thymomas	Follow-up	Complete Remission Rate of MG in Thymomas vs Nonthymomas
Papatestas et al,[42] 1987	174	10 y	10% thymomas vs 24% nonthymomas
Maggi et al,[14] 1989	162	5–10 y	15.7% thymomas vs 37.9% nonthymomas
Evoli et al,[13] 2002	207	Mean 10.1 y	9.2% for thymomas
López-Cano et al,[55] 2003	108	Mean 10 y (9 mo–33 y)	16% for thymomas
Lucchi et al,[54] 2009	123	Mean 76 mo	5 y, 43%; 10 y, 47% (Kaplan-Meier) for thymomas
Maggi et al,[16] 2008	197	Mean 7.69 ± 6 y	9.64% for thymomas

reached complete remission. These results that are based on the analysis of the European population are considerably different from those of Asian studies.

RECURRENCE OF THYMOMA

Recurrence of thymoma is localized almost always inside the chest, in the mediastinum, or intrapleurally.[62,63] The mean time interval between thymectomy and recurrence was 86 months (4–192 months),[63] 88 months (29–306 months),[62] and 8.76 ± 5.5 years (2.7–28.0 years).[16] Presence of MG did not affect recurrence proportion, disease-free interval, or survival after recurrence.[63]

According to Evoli and colleagues,[13] there were no recurrences in patients with stage I or in patients with types A and AB thymomas. The time to recurrence was shorter for more advanced tumors (the mean time interval between thymectomy and recurrence was 8.5 years for stage II, 5.8 years for stage III, and 3.25 years for stage IVA). The rate of recurrence reported by Maggi and colleagues[16] was 9.6%, with only 1 of 19 patients achieving complete stable remission. Regarding the WHO classification of histologic types, the recurrence rate was 8.9% in type AB, 17.2% in type B1, 9.8% in type B2, 28.6% in types B2 and B3, and 5.6% in type B3; no recurrences were found in type A. The recurrence rate according to the Masaoka staging is as follows: stage I, 0; stage II-1, 27.6%; stage II-2, 7.7%; and stage III, 17.4%. Time to thymoma recurrence was independent from the Masaoka stage. Monden and

colleagues[64] and Nakahara and colleagues[65] found recurrence rate in patients with MG-associated thymoma versus patients with non-MG thymoma, even in cases with similar clinical stages. Kondo and Monden[12] described results of treatment of 1089 patients with thymoma from 115 surgical departments operated on in the period from 1990 to 1994 in Japan. There was an association between MG and thymomas in 24.8% of patients. The recurrence rates in both groups were not different, which were 6.4% in MG-associated group versus 8.3% in the group without MG. In patients with MG, the number of stage IVB tumors was lower (15% vs 34%) and the resectability was higher (60% vs 38%) when compared to the group without MG.

MORTALITY AND MORBIDITY IN PATIENTS WITH THYMOMAS ASSOCIATED WITH MG, AUTOIMMUNE DISEASES, AND SECOND MALIGNANCY

MG and recurrence of thymoma are the 2 most important causes of death during follow-up of patients with MG associated with thymoma (**Table 5**). In 5% to 10% of patients, thymoma is accompanied by an autoimmune disease syndrome other than MG, including pure red cell aplasia, hypogammaglobulinemia (about 2%–5% each), and other less common syndromes.[18] About 4% to 7% of patients with thymoma and MG have more than 1 paraneoplastic syndrome.[19]

During the mean follow-up period of 10.1 years, other autoimmune diseases were diagnosed in 9.7% and in 10% of patients.[14] Thymoma

Table 5
Rates of deaths of patients operated on for thymoma with associated MG

Authors	No. of Patients	Duration of Follow-up	Rate of Deaths Caused By MG (%)	Rate of Deaths Caused By Tumor Recurrence (%)
Evoli et al,[13] 2002	207	Mean 10.1 y	3.9	3.4
Maggi et al,[16] 2008	197	Mean 7.69 ± 6 y	1.5	5.6
Margaritora et al,[19] 2010	276	144.7 ± 104.4 mo	3.3	5.4
López-Cano et al,[55] 2003	108	Mean 10 y (9 mo–33 y)	13.0	5.6
Okumura et al,[21] 2002	127	Mean 11.3 ± 7.8 y	11.0	10.3

increases the risk of second malignancy. According to Maggi and colleagues,[16] 11.1% of patients developed extrathymic malignancies. According to Owe and colleagues,[66] extrathymic malignancies occurred in 10% of patients with thymoma during the 10 years after thymoma diagnosis. The risk was significantly increased compared with general population. Thymoma morphology was not a significant predictor for an increased risk of consecutive cancer occurrence. There is no specific type of cancer linked with thymoma. The risk of extrathymic malignancies was similar in patients with MG associated thymoma and non-MG thymoma. The immunologic process underlying MG has no influence on the risk of cancer in patients with thymoma. Evoli and colleagues[67] compared patients with thymoma with and without MG for incidence of extrathymic malignancies. They found a significantly higher rate of additional tumors in patients without MG. According to the investigators' opinion, these findings could be related to an apparent protective effect of MG in thymomas.

SUMMARY

There are several conclusions that can be made about MG associated with thymomas. This type of MG differs from nonthymomatous MG. Probably, pathomechanisms of both types of MG are not the same. Thymomas associated with MG are also different from non-MG thymomas. Patients with thymoma-associated MG tend to be significantly younger than those with non-MG thymoma. Mean duration of MG from the onset of symptoms to thymectomy was significantly shorter than nonthymomatous MG. According to the WHO classification, the incidence of MG in thymomas was the highest in the subtypes B2, B1, and AB. Antititin and antiryanodine receptor

antibodies are found in up to 95% of patients with MG with thymoma, which is much more frequent than in those with nonthymomatous MG. The basis of treatment of thymomas is complete removal of the tumor. Transsternal approach is still regarded the gold standard for surgical treatment of thymomas. Less invasive techniques of thymectomy are promising, but it is too early to estimate the real oncological value of these approaches. For the series including more than 100 patients, the prognosis for survival in patients with thymomas associated with MG is better than those with non-MG thymomas, and the prognosis for patients with MG associated with thymoma is worse than those with nonthymomatous MG. Recurrence of thymoma is localized almost always inside the chest, in the mediastinum, or intrapleurally. The mean time interval between thymectomy and recurrence was 86 to 105 months. Presence of MG did not affect recurrence proportion, disease-free interval, or survival after recurrence. Extrathymic malignancies occurred in 10% of patients with thymoma during the 10 years after thymoma diagnosis. The risk was significantly increased compared with general population. Thymoma morphology was not a significant predictor for an increased risk of consecutive cancer occurrence. There is no specific type of cancer linked with thymoma. The risk of extrathymic malignancies was similar in patients with MG-associated thymoma and non-MG thymoma.

REFERENCES

1. Rosai J, Sobin L. Histological typing of tumors of the thymus. New York. In: World Health Organization, International Histological Classification of Tumors 2nd edition. Berlin: Springer; 1999. p. 9–14.

2. Kirchner T, Muller-Hermelink HK. New approaches to the diagnosis of thymic epithelial tumors. Progr Surg Pathol 1989;10:167–89.

3. Suster S, Rosai L. Thymic carcinoma: a clinopathologic study of 60 cases. Cancer 1991;67:1025–32.

4. Blumberg D, Burt ME, Bains MS, et al. Thymic carcinoma. Ten years experience in twenty patients. J Thorac Cardiovasc Surg 1994;107:615–20.

5. Detterbeck F, Parsons A. Thymic tumors. Ann Thorac Surg 2004;77:1860–9.

6. Johnson S, Eng T, Giaccone G, et al. Thymoma: update for the new millenium. Oncologist 2001;6:239–46.

7. Ströbel P, Preisshofen T, Helmreich M, et al. Pathomechanisms of paraneoplastic myasthenia gravis. Clin Dev Immunol 2003;10(1):7–12.

8. Engels EA, Pfeiffer RM. Malignant thymoma in the United States: demographic patterns in incidence and associations with subsequent malignancies. Int J Cancer 2003;105:546–51.

9. Somnier F. Exacerbation of myasthenia gravis after removal of thymoma. Acta Neurol Scand 1994;90:56–66.

10. Teoh R, McGuire L, Wong K, et al. Increased incidence of thymoma in Chinese myasthenia gravis: possible relationship with Epstein-Barr virus. Acta Neurol Scand 1989;80:221–5.

11. Chiu HC, Vincent A, Newson-Davis J, et al. Myasthenia gravis: population differences in disease expression and acetylcholine receptor antibody titers between Chinese and Caucasian. Neurology 1987;37:1854–7.

12. Kondo K, Monden Y. Thymoma and myasthenia gravis: a clinical study of 1,089 patients from Japan. Ann Thorac Surg 2005;79:219–24.

13. Evoli A, Minisci C, Di Schino C, et al. Thymoma in patients with MG. Neurology 2002;59:1844–50.

14. Maggi G, Casadio C, Cavallo R, et al. Thymectomy in myasthenia gravis. Results of 662 cases operated upon in 15 years. Eur J Cardiothorac Surg 1989;3:504–11.

15. Masaoka A, Yamakawa Y, Niwa H, et al. Extended thymectomy for myasthenia gravis patients: a 20-year review. Ann Thorac Surg 1996;62:853–9.

16. Maggi L, Andreetta F, Antozzi C, et al. Thymoma-associated myasthenia gravis: outcome, clinical and pathological correlations in 197 patients on a 20-year experience. J Neuroimmunol 2008;201–202:237–44.

17. Osserman KE, Genkins G. Studies in myasthenia gravis: review of a twenty-year experience in over 1200 patients. Mt Sinai J Med 1971;38:497–537.

18. Jaretzki A, Barohn R, Ernstoff R, et al. Task force of the Medical Scientific Advisory Board of the Myasthenia Gravis Foundation of America. Myasthenia gravis: recommendations for clinical research standards. Ann Thorac Surg 2000;70:327–34.

19. Margaritora S, Casario A, Cusumano G, et al. Thirty-five year follow-up analysis of clinical and pathologic outcomes of thymoma surgery. Ann Thorac Surg 2010;89:245–52.

20. Chen G, Marx A, Wen-Hu C, et al. New WHO histologic classification predicts prognosis of thymic epithelial tumors: a clinicopathologic study of 200 thymoma cases from China. Cancer 2002;95(2):420–9.

21. Okumura M, Ohta M, Tateyama H, et al. The World Health Organization histologic classification system reflects the oncologic behavior of thymoma. Cancer 2002;94:624–32.

22. Romi F, Gilhus N, Varhaug J, et al. Disease severity and outcome in thymoma myasthenia gravis: a long-term observation study. Eur J Neurol 2003;10:701–6.

23. Romi F, Bø L, Skeie GO, et al. Titin and ryanodine receptor epitopes are expressed in cortical thymoma along with costimulatory molecules. J Neuroimmunol 2002;128:82–9.

24. Kondo K, Monden Y. Therapy for thymic epithelial tumors: a clinical study of 1,320 patients from Japan. Ann Thorac Surg 2003;76:878–85.

25. Mangi A, Wright C, Allan J, et al. Adjuvant radiation therapy for stage II thymoma. Ann Thorac Surg 2002;74:1037.

26. Mangi A, Wain J, Donahue D, et al. Adjuvant radiation of stage III thymoma. Ann Thorac Surg 2005;79:1834–9.

27. Kondo K, Moden Y. Myasthenia gravis appearing after thymectomy for thymoma. Eur J Cardiothorac Surg 2005;28:22–5.

28. Regnard JF, Magdeleinat P, Dromer C, et al. Prognostic factors and long-term results after thymoma resection: a series of 307 patients. J Thorac Cardiovasc Surg 1996;112:376–84.

29. Toker A, Tanju S, Ozluk Y, et al. Thymoma appearing 10 years after an extended thymectomy for myasthenia gravis. Eur J Cardiothorac Surg 2008;33(6):1155–6.

30. Awad W, Symmans P, Dussek J. Recurrence of stage thymoma 32 years after total excision. Ann Thorac Surg 1998;66:2106–8.

31. Hirabayashi H, Ohta M, Okumura M, et al. Appearance of thymoma 15 years after extended thymectomy for myasthenia gravis without thymoma. Eur J Cardiothorac Surg 2002;22:479–81.

32. Ruckert J, Walter M, Muller J. Pulmonary function after thoracoscopic thymectomy versus median sternotomy for myasthenia gravis. Ann Thorac Surg 2000;70:1656–61.

33. Shigemura N, Shiono H, Inoue M, et al. Inclusion of the transcervical approach in video-assisted thoracoscopic extended thymectomy (VATET) for myasthenia gravis: a prospective trial. Surg Endosc 2006;20(10):1614–8.

34. Cooper J. Video-assisted thoracic surgery for myasthenia gravis: commentary. Chest Surg Clin N Am 1998;8:827–33.

35. Yim A, Kay R, Izaat M, et al. Video-assisted thoracoscopic thymectomy for myasthenia gravis. Semin Thorac Cardiovasc Surg 1999;11:65–73.

36. Savcenko M, Wendt G, Prince S, et al. Video-assisted thymectomy for myasthenia gravis: an update of a single institution experience. Eur J Cardiothorac Surg 2002;22(6):978–83.

37. Mineo T, Pompeo E, Lerut T, et al. Thoracoscopic thymectomy in autoimmune myasthenia: results of left-sided approach. Ann Thorac Surg 2000;69:1537–41.

38. Roviaro G, Varoli F, Nucca O, et al. Videothoracoscopic approach to primary mediastinal pathology. Chest 2000;117:1179–83.

39. Takeo S, Sakada T, Yano T. Video-assisted extended thymectomy in patients with thymoma by lifting the sternum. Ann Thorac Surg 2001;71:1721–3.

40. Ohta M, Hirabayasi H, Okumura M, et al. Thoracoscopic thymectomy using anterior chest wall lifting method. Ann Thorac Surg 2003;76:1310–1.

41. Hsu C, Chuang C, Hsu N, et al. Comparison between the right side and subxiphoid bilateral approaches in performing video-assisted thoracoscopic extended thymectomy for myasthenia gravis. Surg Endosc 2004;18:821–4.

42. Papatestas AE, Pozner J, Genkins G. Prognosis in occult thymomas in myasthenia gravis following trancervical thymectomy. Arch Surg 1987;122:1352–6.

43. Deeb M, Brinster C, Kucharzuk J, et al. Expanded indications for transcervical thymectomy in the management of anterior mediastinal masses. Ann Thorac Surg 2001;72:208–11.

44. Odaka M, Akiba T, Yabe M, et al. Unilateral thoracoscopic subtotal thymectomy for the treatment of stage I and II thymoma. Eur J Cardiothorac Surg 2010;37:824–6.

45. Cheng YJ, Kao EL, Chou SH. Videothoracoscopic resection of stage II thymoma: prospective comparison of the results between thoracoscopy and open methods. Chest 2005;128:3010–2.

46. Soon JL, Agasthian T. Harmonic scalpel in video-assisted thoracoscopic thymic resections. Asian Cardiovasc Thorac Ann 2008;16:366–9.

47. Agasthian T, Lin SJ. Clinical outcome of video-assisted thymectomy for myasthenia gravis and thymoma. Asian Cardiovasc Thorac Ann 2010;18:234–9.

48. Uchiyama A, Shimizu S, Murai H, et al. Infrasternal mediastinoscopic surgery for anterior mediastinal masses. Surg Endosc 2004;18(5):843–6.

49. Sakamaki Y, Kido T, Yasukawa M. Alternative choices of total and partial thymectomy in video-assisted resection of noninvasive thymomas. Surg Endosc 2008;22(5):1272–7.

50. Augustin F, Schmid T, Sieb M, et al. Video-assisted thoracoscopic surgery versus robotic-assisted thoracoscopic surgery thymectomy. Ann Thorac Surg 2008;85(2):S768–71.

51. Savitt M, Gao G, Furnary A, et al. Application of robotic-assisted techniques to the surgical evaluation and treatment of the anterior mediastinum. Ann Thorac Surg 2005;79:450–5.

52. Rückert JC, Swierzy M, Rückert RI, et al. Benefits and limits of minimally invasive surgery for thymic tumors. Abstract T13. Annual Meeting of the International Society for Minimally Invasive Cardiothoracic Burgery (ISMICS) [abstract book]. Berlin, June 16–19, 2010.

53. Ponseti JM, Gamez J, Azem J, et al. Post-thymectomy combined treatment of prednisone and tacrolimus versus prednisone alone for consolidation of complete stable remission in patients with myasthenia gravis: a non-randomized, non-controlled study. Curr Med Res Opin 2007;23(6):1269–78.

54. Lucchi M, Ricciardi R, Melfi F, et al. Association of thymoma and myasthenia gravis: oncological and neurological results of the surgical treatment. Eur J Cardiothorac Surg 2009;35(5):812–6.

55. López-Cano M, Ponseti-Bosch JM, Espin-Basany E, et al. Clinical and pathologic predictors of outcome in thymoma-associated myasthenia gravis. Ann Thorac Surg 2003;76(5):1643–9.

56. Hsu H, Huang C, Huang B, et al. Thymoma is associated with relapse of symptoms after transsternal thymectomy for myasthenia gratis. Interact Cardiovasc Thorac Surg 2006;5:42–6.

57. Tsinzerling N, Lefvert AK, Matell G, et al. Myasthenia gravis: a long term follow-up study of Swedish patients with specific reference to thymic histology. J Neurol Neurosurg Psychiatr 2007;78:1109–12.

58. Namba T, Brunner NG, Grob D. Myasthenia gravis in patients with thymoma, with particular reference to onset after thymectomy. Medicine (Baltimore) 1978;57:411–33.

59. Ito M, Fujimura S, Monden Y, et al. [A retrospective group study on post-thymectomy myasthenia gravis]. Nippon Kyobu Geka Gakkai Zasshi 1992;19:189–93 [in Japanese].

60. Nakajima J, Murakawa T, Fukami T, et al. Postthymectomy myasthenia gravis: relationship with thymoma and antiacetylcholine receptor antibody. Ann Thorac Surg 2008;86:941–5.

61. Tseng YL, Chang JM, Shu IL, et al. Myasthenia gravis developed 30 months after resection of recurrent thymoma. Eur J Cardiothorac Surg 2006;29(2):268.

62. Regnard JF, Zinzindohoue F, Magdeleinat P, et al. Results of re-resection for recurrent thymomas. Ann Thorac Surg 1997;64:1593–8.

63. Ruffini E, Manusco M, Oliaro A, et al. Recurrence of thymoma: analysis of clinocopathologic features,

treatment, and outcome. J Thorac Cardiovasc Surg 1997;113:55–63.

64. Monden Y, Nakahara K, Iioka S, et al. Recurrence of thymoma: clinicopathological features, therapy, and prognosis. Ann Thorac Surg 1985;39:165–9.

65. Nakahara K, Ohno K, Hashimoto J, et al. Thymoma: results with complete resection and adjuvant postoperative irradiation in 141 consecutive patients. J Thorac Cardiovasc Surg 1988;95: 1041–7.

66. Owe J, Cvancarova M, Romi F, et al. Extrathymic malignancies in thymoma patients with and without myasthenia gravis. J Neurol Sci 2010;290:66–9.

67. Evoli A, Punzi C, Marsili F, et al. Extrathymic malignancies in patients with thymoma. Ann Oncol 2004;15: 692–3.

68. Okumura M, Miyoshi S, Takeuchi Y, et al. Results of surgical treatment of thymomas with special reference to the involved organs. J Thorac Cardiovasc Surg 1999;117:605–11.

Management of Stage I and II Thymoma

Frank C. Detterbeck, MD[a],*, Alden M. Parsons, MD[b]

KEYWORDS

- Thymoma • Surgery • Radiation • Evaluation
- Clinical presentation • Recurrence

Thymoma is a relatively rare disease, and other anterior mediastinal tumors are even more uncommon. Being able to make the correct clinical diagnosis is important, because management of other anterior mediastinal tumors is quite different. Because these patients often present at many different institutions, where there is often only limited experience with mediastinal tumors, often there is lack of a structured approach to these patients. This article provides a framework for how to approach these patients.

For thymoma, appropriate treatment has a very high rate of cure. Often there is a lack of appreciation for the fact that all thymomas are malignant. Furthermore, there is often confusion about what constitutes appropriate care, and patients end up with incomplete resection, debulking procedures, and unnecessary adjuvant treatment. If this occurs, an opportunity for an excellent result from treatment has thus been squandered. This article reviews the data regarding the treatment of early-stage thymoma.

EVALUATION
Clinical Presentation

Of all patients with thymoma, approximately 30% are asymptomatic, 40% present with local symptoms related to the intrathoracic mass, and approximately 30% have systemic symptoms. A review of studies[1] reporting details of the clinical presentations leads to several conclusions. Chest pain, cough, and dyspnea are the most common symptoms. Superior vena cava (SVC) syndrome

and weight loss do occur in a small proportion of patients, although such symptoms are generally associated with more aggressive tumors. Finally, a small proportion of patients present with a fever or night sweats, which are more typically associated with lymphoma.

Thymomas are often associated with a variety of conditions called "parathymic syndromes,"[2,3] which, if present, clearly point the diagnosis of an anterior mediastinal mass toward thymoma. The most common associated syndrome is myasthenia gravis (MG), which occurs in approximately 45% of patients with thymoma among larger studies.[1] Conversely, only approximately 10% to 15% of patients with MG are found to have a thymoma, although among patients with MG who undergo thymectomy, approximately 25% have a thymoma.[1] MG is widely recognized to be an autoimmune disease, characterized in most patients by antibodies that cross-react between the thymus and the acetylcholine receptor in the neuromuscular endplate.[4] However, it is unclear how a thymoma causes MG or vice versa.[4] Patients with MG commonly present with ptosis, double vision, or generalized fatigue, particularly worse late in the day. Other parathymic syndromes are seen in approximately 6% of patients with thymoma. These are also autoimmune processes, especially hypogammaglobunlinemia and pure red cell dyscrasia.

The gender distribution of thymoma is approximately equal, although it is slightly more common in women in older age groups. Thymomas occur in all ages, but there is a broad peak between approximately 40 to 70 years.[1] Patients with MG

[a] Section of Thoracic Surgery, Yale University School of Medicine, PO Box 208062, New Haven, CT 06520-8062, USA
[b] Thoracic Surgery, Rex Thoracic Specialists, 2800 Blue Ridge Road, Suite 403, Raleigh, NC 27607, USA
* Corresponding author.
E-mail address: frank.detterbeck@yale.edu

Thorac Surg Clin 21 (2011) 59–67
doi:10.1016/j.thorsurg.2010.08.001

thoracic.theclinics.com

tend to be slightly younger, with a broad peak between 30 and 60 years.[1]

Radiographic Appearance

Thymomas are the most common cause of an anterior mediastinal mass, accounting for approximately 50% overall.[5–7] The differential diagnosis of anterior mediastinal masses includes thymic tumors, lymphomas, germ cell tumors, thyroid goiters, duplication cysts, and a variety of other less common tumors. Lymphoma accounts for approximately 25% of anterior mediastinal masses, with Hodgkin lymphoma being more common than non-Hodgkin lymphoma.[5–7]

Each of these tumors has radiographic features that help to distinguish it from others. Thymomas typically appear as a well-defined, round, or oval mass in the anterior mediastinum within or involving the normal bed of the thymus gland.[8] They are generally anterior to the great vessels and the heart, but many larger thymomas drape around the great vessels toward either the right or left pulmonary hilum.[9] Calcification may be seen in approximately 10% to 20% of patients, and is typically curvilinear.[8,10–12] Mediastinal lymphomas typically present with enlargement of multiple lymph nodes, including paratracheal, subcarinal, hilar, and periesophageal nodes (which would be very atypical for thymoma).[8] Thyroid masses are generally easily and reliably recognized by a characteristic radiographic appearance (high density), continuity with the thyroid gland, and extension posterior to the great vessels.[8] Malignant germ cell tumors are often large, inhomogeneous, and lobulated. The radiographic appearance of teratomas is often quite characteristic, with cystic areas and mixed areas of calcification and fat.[8] However, the radiographic features of mediastinal tumors are usually only sufficient in generating a strong suspicion of a particular diagnosis, but making a treatment decision requires that one is quite certain. Therefore, other clinical factors and tests must be taken into consideration.

Clinical Approach to Patient Evaluation

The presence of a parathymic condition such as MG and an anterior mediastinal mass is essentially pathognomonic for a thymoma. Thymoma accounts for 50% of anterior mediastinal masses in patients older than 50, and 70% if substernal goiters are excluded, which are usually easy to recognize. In this age group one can be quite certain that a mass that has a typical appearance of a thymoma is, in fact, a thymoma. Difficulty arises primarily in the 20- to 40-year-old group.

In women of this age lymphoma accounts for approximately 50% of anterior mediastinal masses; in men the diagnoses are mixed. Fortunately, most thymomas in this age group have MG and an indolent presentation, whereas most lymphomas have typical symptoms of fevers, night sweats, and with a rapid progression of symptoms. A rapid onset of symptoms points toward lymphoma or a malignant germ cell tumor. Finally, thymomas are relatively uncommon in those younger than 20. These clinical features are generally sufficient to guide the approach to further evaluation.

In patients with MG or in an older age group with a typical radiographic appearance and presentation, one can be quite certain of the diagnosis of thymoma. These patients do not need a biopsy to confirm the diagnosis, and surgical resection based on clinical diagnosis alone is justified. Frozen section confirmation at the time of resection is difficult at best, and should not be used unless unexpected findings are encountered intraoperatively.[13] In younger patients with a presentation suggesting lymphoma, a biopsy to confirm this diagnosis is indicated (often a needle biopsy will yield insufficient material and surgical biopsy is necessary). In the 20- to 40-year-old group, especially men with a rapid onset of symptoms, serum α-fetoprotein (α-FP) and β-human chorionic gonadotrophin (β-HCG) levels should be assessed, as these are elevated in more than 90% of nonseminomatous germ cell tumors.[5] Pursuing these blood tests in other age groups is nonproductive (the incidence of such tumors is <1%) unless there are unusual features to make one suspect a germ cell tumor. In seminomas, β-HCG is elevated in about 10%, and α-FP is normal. If the presentation and blood tests do not suggest another diagnosis (and typically a confirmatory biopsy) and a thymoma is suspected (although there is no MG or parathymic condition), a confirmatory biopsy is generally indicated.

There is no harm in performing a needle or incisional biopsy of a thymoma, if neccessary.[14] Spread of tumor as a result of a biopsy has not been found to occur, despite an earlier concern that this might be the case. Furthermore, no adverse effects have been noted in many centers with extensive experience in thymoma in which it has been standard policy to obtain a biopsy of larger thymomas.[15–21]

The sensitivity of a needle biopsy is about 60% and that of a surgical biopsy about 90%.[1] The ability to accurately determine the histologic type of thymoma on a limited biopsy is limited because of variability within the tumor and other difficulties related to histologic classification.[22–24]

Thymoma Clinical Staging

A major prognostic factor in thymoma is the tumor stage, and this is a major determinant in selecting the best treatment. Although thymoma is not addressed in the Stage Classification Handbook, the Masaoka-Koga classification system (**Table 1**) is most commonly used and has been adopted as the standard by the International Thymic Malignancy Interest Group (ITMIG).[25] The distinction between stage II and III is that the latter invades adjacent mediastinal structures such as the lung, innominate vein, or pericardium of great vessels. This distinction is important, as generally stage I or II thymoma is treated with surgical resection, whereas stage III or IVa thymoma is treated with preoperative chemotherapy before resection.

The Masaoka-Koga staging system addresses the pathologic stage, and little work has been done to define how reliable preoperative clinical staging is and what criteria it should be based on. In a presentation at the 2010 ITMIG, it was reported that stage I and II could be distinguished from higher stages by tumor size, tumor homogeneity, border, lobulation, fat infiltration, and more than 50% abutment of vessels ($P<.02$). Stage I and IIb could be distinguished from higher stage by border margination ($P = .002$) and more than 50% abutment of vessels ($P = .02$).[26] In a small series of 15 patients with a thymoma in which the fat planes between the tumor and adjacent structures were only partially preserved, the sensitivity of this finding in demonstrating invasion was only 53%.[27] Another study found that the impression of invasion into adjacent structures carried a false positive rate of 20% (1 of 5), and the impression of an absence of invasion carried a false negative rate of 7% (1 of 15).[28]

An additional distinction is between thymoma and thymic carcinoma, as thymic carcinoma has a significantly worse prognosis and often an advanced presentation not amenable to complete surgical resection. Radiographic differentiation between thymoma and thymic carcinoma has been addressed in one study of 53 patients.[12] The CT characteristics that were most helpful in predicting that a thymic tumor is *not* a well-differentiated or undifferentiated thymic carcinoma were (1) a smooth or lobulated (not irregular) contour (false positive rate [FP] 13%, false negative rate [FN] 41%, sensitivity 89%, specificity 54%), (2) homogeneous enhancement (FP 6%, FN 51%, sensitivity 74%, specificity 83%), and (3) the absence of any areas of low attenuation (FP 13%, FN 65%, sensitivity 63%, specificity 67%). The characteristics that best predicted the presence of either a routine thymoma or a well-differentiated thymic carcinoma (and not an undifferentiated thymic carcinoma) were (1) a smooth or lobulated contour (FP 5%, FN 45%, sensitivity 88%, specificity 75%), (2) homogeneous enhancement (FP 3%, FN 65%, sensitivity 70%, specificity 88%), (3) the absence of any areas of low attenuation (FP 10%, FN 78%, sensitivity 60%, specificity 63%), (4) the absence of a pleural or pericardial effusion (FP 5%, FN 33%, sensitivity 93%, specificity 75%), and (5) the absence of any calcification (FP 3%, FN 78%, sensitivity 98%, specificity 45%).[12]

TREATMENT
Surgical Resection

Surgical resection has been the mainstay of treatment of thymoma, with a reported operative mortality of 2% and a complication rate of approximately 20%.[1] The 10-year overall survival rates are approximately 90% and 70% for stage I and II, and 55% and 35% for stage III and IVa thymoma

Table 1
Masaoka-Koga staging system

Stage	Definition
I	Grossly and microscopically completely encapsulated tumor
II a	Microscopic transcapsular invasion
b	Macroscopic invasion into thymic or surrounding fatty tissue, or grossly adherent to but not breaking through mediastinal pleura or pericardium
III	Macroscopic invasion into neighboring organ (ie, pericardium, great vessel or lung)
IV a	Pleural or pericardial metastases
b	Lymphogenous or hematogenous metastasis

From Koga K, Matsuno Y, Noguchi M, et al. A review of 79 thymomas: modification of staging system and reappraisal of conventional division into invasive and non-invasive thymoma. Pathol Int 1994;44(5):359–67.

(Fig. 1).[1] However, only a very small fraction of deaths in stage I or II thymoma are attributable to thymoma. Therefore, the ITMIG consensus is that freedom from recurrence is probably a better measure,[25] although data for this are limited at this point. The reported recurrence rates from multiple studies are 3%, 11%, 30%, and 43% in resected stage I, II, III, and IVa thymoma (but these are not actuarial rates at a particular point in time).[1] An approximation of actuarial recurrence is the disease-free survival, which is approximately 94% and 88% for stage I and II, and 56% and 33% for stage III and IVa thymoma at 10 years.[1]

Extent of resection

Significantly better survival has been noted in patients who underwent complete resection by every large study examining this issue.[15,16,29-37] Among completely resected patients, the 10-year overall survival is 80%, 78%, 75%, and 42% for stages I, II, III, and IVa, respectively.[29] Other studies have also demonstrated good survival after complete resection in patients with a stage III or IV thymoma.[38] It is remarkable that the long-term survival of patients with a stage III thymoma is similar to that of those with a stage I thymoma, provided a complete resection was able to be performed. These findings imply that the ability to carry out a complete resection may be the most important factor. This was also noted in a multivariate analysis of 307 patients, in which a complete resection was the only significant prognostic factor (stage was not significant if completeness of resection was included in the model).[29]

Many centers with a large experience with thymomas recommend that a complete thymectomy be done, even if only a portion of the thymus is involved with a thymoma.[15,29,32,39-44] However,

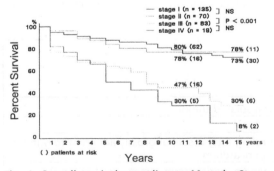

Fig. 1. Overall survival according to Masaoka Stage. NS, not significant. (*From* Regnard J-F, Magdeleinat P, Dromer C, et al. Prognostic factors and long-term results after thymoma resection: a series of 307 patients. J Thorac Cardiovasc Surg 1996;112:376–84; with permission.)

there are few data to either substantiate or refute this. A second small thymoma was found in 3% of 264 patients undergoing thymectomy for thymoma in one large study.[29] The occasional occurrence of multicentric thymomas has been corroborated in several other studies.[10,43,45,46] In addition, anecdotal cases of occurrence of myasthenia several years after incomplete thymectomy in previously asymptomatic patients have been reported,[43,47–50] although it is not clear that this can be prevented by a complete thymectomy. Better survival after complete thymectomy (n = 16) compared with tumor resection alone (n = 18) was suggested in one study that has analyzed this (5-year survival 92% vs 59%, $P<.05$ at that point in time; 10-year survival 47% vs 44%).[41] However, another study suggested no difference in survival after complete thymectomy (n = 71) compared with tumor resection alone (n = 55).[51]

Approaches

Most institutions with experience in this field favor a sternotomy as the optimal incision in patients with a thymoma[15,18,29,39–44] with few exceptions.[16,20,37] This is consistent with the recommendation for complete thymectomy, as it is difficult to perform a complete thymectomy through a thoracotomy.[39] Incisions other than a median sternotomy are occasionally used, including a transcervical approach.[52–54]

Minimally invasive (thoracoscopic, transcervical, and robotic) approaches to early stage thymomas have recently been explored. However, because long-term data are not yet available, and because preoperative imaging characteristics have been poorly studied, this approach should probably be avoided at this point except in centers with extensive experience. A complete resection is achieved in virtually all patients with a stage I and II thymoma using open techniques. Whether this is true for minimally invasive approaches is not yet clear. The ITMIG organization is defining standards for minimally invasive resection of thymoma.

Adjuvant Therapy

There is little or no role for adjuvant chemotherapy in stage I and II thymoma. Whether adjuvant radiotherapy should be given after a resection has been controversial. Some investigators have recommended this for all patients, regardless of stage or completeness of resection,[32,55] others for only stage II and III thymomas[20,29,39,47,56–58] or for incompletely resected patients.[47,56,59–61] Although the vast majority of recurrences of a thymoma are local, most of these local recurrences involve pleural or pericardial implants that are not necessarily contiguous with the original tumor location.[34]

Several reviews and meta-analyses of individual reports have now consistently demonstrated no benefit to postoperative radiotherapy (RT) in completely resected stage I and II thymoma (**Fig. 2**).[1,14,59–62] It should be noted, however, that these series are not based on randomized patients. In incompletely resected patients, a stronger argument for adjuvant RT can be made, based on a stronger rationale and some limited data. However, in stage I and II thymoma, an incomplete resection is extremely rare.

RECURRENCE
Recurrence Pattern

Tumors of the thymus that show no cytologic features of malignancy *and* show no gross evidence of invasion have sometimes been called "benign" thymomas.[41,42,47,63] However, despite the indolent behavior of such tumors, recurrences and metastases have been reported in all large series following resection,[15,29,36,64–66] making this is a misleading term. This is true even for stage I thymomas,[15,29–33,35,36,51,55,65–69] and is true for each histologic subtype of thymoma.[29,32,33,51,65,69–71] Only a few smaller series

did not observe recurrences among smaller cohorts of patients with medullary thymomas[21,64,72,73] or type A thymomas.[36,74–76] Thus, even cytologically bland thymomas have the fundamental characteristics of a malignant tumor (ability to invade tissues and metastasize). Because the natural history of the tumor is one of rather slow growth, and because an effective treatment is available (resection) does not alter this fact. Therefore, all thymomas are, in fact, malignant, and the term "benign thymoma" should be discarded.

The indolent behavior of thymic tumors is demonstrated by the average time to recurrence of approximately 4 to 5 years,[15,16,29,33,35,66] with a range from 3 to 4 months[16,33,66] to 10 to 15 years in most studies.[15,16,29,35,66] One study that analyzed this by stage found that the mean time to recurrence was 10 years in patients with a stage I thymoma, compared with 3 years in patients with a stage II to IV thymoma.[65]

Local and regional recurrence is by far more common than a distant recurrence. In the past the term "local recurrence" referred to any recurrence in the thorax, but this usage was too broad and refinement of the terms was needed. The

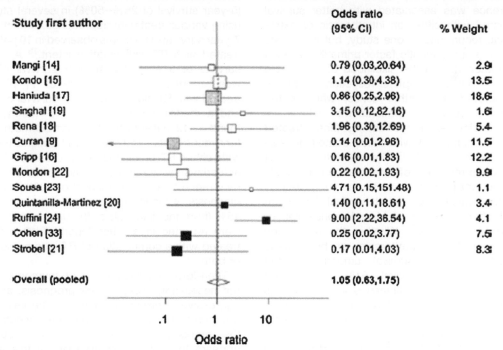

Fig. 2. Role of adjuvant RT. Forest plot generated using extracted recurrence data for patients with stage II and III thymic epithelial tumors. The squares represent the odds ratios of the individual studies, and the size of the squares reflect the calculated weight of the study in the meta-analysis. The horizontal bars running through each square represent the 95% confidence interval (CI). The diamond at the bottom of the plot illustrates the combined odds ratio using a fixed effects model. (White boxes, stage II; gray boxes, stages II and III; black boxes, stage III.) (*From* Korst RJ, Kansler AL, Christos PJ, et al. Adjuvant radiotherapy for thymic epithelial tumors: a systematic review and meta-analysis. Ann Thorac Surg 2009;87(5):1641–7; with permission.)

ITMIG organization has defined local recurrence as a recurrence in the anterior mediastinum (ie, in the location of the normal thymus gland).[25] A regional recurrence is an intrathoracic recurrence not adjacent to the thymus or previous thymoma (ie, pleural or pericardial nodules). A distant recurrence is outside the chest or involving intraparenchymal pulmonary nodules.[25] Using these definitions approximately 25% of recurrences are local, 60% regional, and 10% distant.[1] Liver and bone are the two most common sites of distant metastases.

Treatment of Recurrence

An aggressive approach to recurrence of thymoma has been advocated by several investigators.[15,16,29,38,39,43,66,77,78] Between half and two-thirds of all recurrences were considered to be operable in those series reporting these data.[16,37,66,77,78] Of those patients in whom reoperation was undertaken, a complete resection was able to be accomplished in 62% (range 45%–71%).[37,43,66,77,78]

Which factors are associated with a favorable prognosis in patients with a recurrent thymoma has not been clearly defined. A mediastinal recurrence was associated with better survival compared with either an intrathoracic or extrathoracic recurrence in one study, but it appears that this is a prognostic factor primarily by being a predictor for a higher likelihood of being able to carry out a complete resection.[66] This is corroborated by another series, which noted that there were more patients with a local (ie, intrathoracic) recurrence among those treated surgically compared with those treated nonsurgically (92% vs 67%).[16] The ability to carry out a complete resection of a recurrence is probably an important prognostic factor, as suggested by the observation that good survival has been noted after resection of pleural, pericardial, or pulmonary implants.[77] Whether the recurrence was mediastinal, intrathoracic, or both made no difference in survival among resected patients (5-year survival 51%, 57%, and 46%).[77] Similarly, no difference in survival was noted in 21 patients treated with curative intent RT (7-year survival of 74%, 77%, and 40% for only mediastinal recurrence, intrathoracic recurrence, or both).[78] The original stage of thymoma and the disease-free interval do not appear to be prognostic factors after the appearance of a recurrence,[16] although this appears to be somewhat at odds with the observation that local recurrences are seen somewhat more commonly in patients who originally had a stage I or II thymoma, and pleural, pericardial, or pulmonary implants in patients who originally had a stage III or IV thymoma.[66,77]

The survival of patients with a recurrence appears to be better if surgery is undertaken. In fact, the survival of patients with a recurrence that was resected was the same as the survival of patients without any recurrence in one study (measured from the diagnosis of the original thymoma).[16] However, it is also possible that patients undergoing resection of a recurrence have a good prognosis compared with patients whose recurrence is not resected simply because they are selected on the basis of favorable characteristics. Most of the available data show good survival among completely resected patients (5- and 10-year survival of approximately 70% and 60%[66,77]) as opposed to incompletely resected patients (5- and 10-year survival of approximately 20% and 5%[29,37,66,77]). A second recurrence was observed in only about 20% of patients after a complete resection of a first recurrence in 2 series (mean follow-up of 4 and 5 years after the recurrence.[43,77]

Other treatments for recurrent thymoma have involved radiation or chemotherapy. Reasonable intermediate-term survival has been reported (5-year survival of 25%–50%) in several studies using various treatment approaches. An actuarial 7-year survival of 65% was observed in 10 patients treated with RT with curative intent.[78] A 5-year survival of 53% and a 10-year survival of 0% was reported in another study of 11 patients treated with RT alone.[66] A 5-year survival of 33% and a median survival time of 10 months was found in 12 patients treated with chemotherapy for a recurrence.[79] In a report of 11 patients treated with either RT or chemotherapy, a 42% 5-year actuarial survival rate was noted from the time of recurrence.[15] A 2-year survival of 30% (from the diagnosis of recurrence) and a 7-year survival of 45% (from the diagnosis of the original thymoma) were reported in another report of 12 patients treated with a combination of RT, chemotherapy, or both.[16]

Therefore, the recurrence of thymoma does not necessarily imply a poor prognosis, and an aggressive approach is justified. The key issue appears to be whether a complete resection of the metastases is likely; surgical resection appears to be the best approach if this is the case. Every effort should be made to achieve a complete resection. If it is likely that only an incomplete resection can be accomplished, it is not clear whether surgery is beneficial compared with treatment with RT or chemotherapy.

SUMMARY

Although the approach to mediastinal tumors can seem difficult, with experience one can make a highly reliable clinical diagnosis is many patients. A biopsy is often not needed, but can be done without adverse oncologic effects if needed. Surgery is the mainstay of treatment for stage I and II thymoma. The rate of complete resection is essentially 100% by open techniques, and recurrences are rare. A complete thymectomy via a sternotomy is the standard approach. Adjuvant radiotherapy after a complete resection does not appear to be of benefit. In the rare event of a recurrence, an aggressive approach should be taken with re-resection whenever possible.

REFERENCES

1. Detterbeck F, Parsons AM. Thymic tumors: a review of current diagnosis, classification, and treatment. Thoracic and esophageal surgery. 3rd edition. Philadelphia: Elsevier; 2008. p.1589–614.

2. Souadjian JV, Enriquez P, Silverstein MN, et al. The spectrum of diseases associated with thymoma. Arch Intern Med 1974;134:374–9.

3. Rosenow EC, Hurley BT. Disorders of the thymus. Arch Intern Med 1984;144:763–70.

4. Drachman DB. Myasthenia gravis. N Engl J Med 1994;330(25):1797–810.

5. Davis RJ, Oldham HN Jr, Sabiston DC. Primary cysts and neoplasms of the mediastinum: recent changes in clinical presentation, methods of diagnosis, management, and results. Ann Thorac Surg 1987; 44:229–37.

6. Mullen B, Richardson JD. Primary anterior mediastinal tumors in children and adults. Ann Thorac Surg 1986;42:338–45.

7. Valli M, Fabris GA, Dewar A, et al. Atypical carcinoid tumour of the thymus: a study of eight cases. Histopathology 1994;24:371–5.

8. Boiselle PM. Mediastinal masses. In: McLoud TC, editor. Thoracic radiology: the requisites. St Louis (MO): Mosby; 1998. p. 431–62.

9. Rosado-de-Christenson ML, Galobardes J, Moran CA. Thymoma: radiologic-pathologic correlation. Radiographics 1992;12:151–68.

10. Ellis K, Austin JHM, Jaretzki A III. Radiologic detection of thymoma in patients with myasthenia gravis. AJR Am J Roentgenol 1988;151:873–81.

11. Brown LR, Muhm JR, Gray JE. Radiographic detection of thymoma. AJR Am J Roentgenol 1980;134: 1181–8.

12. Tomiyama N, Johkoh T, Mihara N, et al. Using the World Health Organization classification of thymic epithelial neoplasms to describe CT findings. AJR Am J Roentgenol 2002;179(4):881–6.

13. ITMIG. Which Way is Up? A collaborative position paper on standards of handling and processing of thymic tissue by surgeons and pathologists. JTO 2010.

14. Detterbeck FC, Parsons AM. Thymic tumors. Ann Thorac Surg 2004;77(5):1860–9.

15. Maggi G, Casadio C, Cavallo A, et al. Thymoma: results of 241 operated cases. Ann Thorac Surg 1991;51:152–6.

16. Blumberg D, Port JL, Weksler B, et al. Thymoma: a multivariate analysis of factors predicting survival. Ann Thorac Surg 1995;60:908–14.

17. Shamji F, Pearson FG, Todd TRJ, et al. Results of surgical treatment for thymoma. J Thorac Cardiovasc Surg 1984;87:43–7.

18. Moore KH, McKenzie PR, Kennedy CW, et al. Thymoma: trends over time. Ann Thorac Surg 2001;72:203–7.

19. Venuta F, Rendina EA, Pescarmona EO, et al. Multimodality treatment of thymoma: a prospective study. Ann Thorac Surg 1997;64:1585–92.

20. Kaiser LR, Martini N. Clinical management of thymomas: the Memorial Sloan-Kettering Cancer Center experience. In: Martini N, Vogt-Moykopf I, editors. Thoracic surgery: frontiers and uncommon neoplasms, vol. 5. St Louis (MO): C V Mosby Co; 1989. p.176–83.

21. Lardinois D, Rechsteiner R, Läng RH, et al. Prognostic relevance of Masaoka and Müller-Hermelink classification in patients with thymic tumors. Ann Thorac Surg 2000;69:1550–5.

22. Moran CA, Suster S. On the histologic heterogeneity of thymic epithelial neoplasms. Impact of sampling in subtyping and classification of thymomas. Am J Clin Pathol 2000;114(5):760–6.

23. Detterbeck FC. Clinical value of the WHO classification system of thymoma. Ann Thorac Surg 2006; 81(6):2328–34.

24. Detterbeck F. Evaluation and treatment of stage I and II thymoma. J Thorac Oncol 2010;5(10):1500–1.

25. Huang J, Wang Z, Loehrer P, et al. Standard outcome measures for thymic malignancies. J Thorac Oncol 2010. [Epub ahead of print].

26. Marom E, Milito M, Moran C, et al. CT findings predicting invasiveness of thymoma [abstract]. J Thorac Oncol 2010. [Epub ahead of print].

27. Chen J, Weisbrod GL, Herman SJ. Computed tomography and pathologic correlations of thymic lesions. J Thorac Imaging 1988;3(1):61–5.

28. Jung K-J, Lee KS, Han J, et al. Malignant thymic epithelial tumors: CT-pathologic correlation. AJR Am J Roentgenol 2001;176:433–9.

29. Regnard J-F, Magdeleinat P, Dromer C, et al. Prognostic factors and long-term results after thymoma resection: a series of 307 patients. J Thorac Cardiovasc Surg 1996;112:376–84.

30. Maggi G, Giaccone G, Donadio M, et al. Thymomas: a review of 169 cases, with particular reference to

results of surgical treatment. Cancer 1986;58: 765–76.

31. Okumura M, Miyoshi S, Takeuchi Y, et al. Results of surgical treatment of thymomas with special reference to the involved organs. J Thorac Cardiovasc Surg 1999;117:605–13.

32. Nakahara K, Ohno K, Hashimoto J, et al. Thymoma: results with complete resection and adjuvant postoperative irradiation in 141 consecutive patients. J Thorac Cardiovasc Surg 1988;95:1041–7.

33. Lewis JE, Wick MR, Scheithauer BW, et al. Thymoma: a clinicopathologic review. Cancer 1987;60: 2727–43.

34. Myojin M, Choi NC, Wright CD, et al. Stage III thymoma: pattern of failure after surgery and postoperative radiotherapy and its implication for future study. Int J Radiat Oncol Biol Phys 2000;46(4):927–33.

35. Wilkins KB, Sheikh E, Green R, et al. Clinical and pathologic predictors of survival in patients with thymoma. Ann Surg 1999;230(4):562–74.

36. Okumura M, Ohta M, Tateyama H, et al. The World Health Organization histologic classification system reflects the oncologic behavior of thymoma: a clinical study of 273 patients. Cancer 2002;94(3):624–32.

37. Rea F, Marulli G, Girardi R, et al. Long-term survival and prognostic factors in thymic epithelial tumours. Eur J Cardiothorac Surg 2004;26(2):412–8.

38. Yagi K, Hirata T, Fukuse T, et al. Surgical treatment for invasive thymoma, especially when the superior vena cava is invaded. Ann Thorac Surg 1996;61: 521–4.

39. Wilkins EJ, Grillo HC, Scannell JG, et al. Role of staging in prognosis and management of thymoma. Ann Thorac Surg 1991;51:888–92.

40. Crucitti F, Doglietto GB, Bellantone R, et al. Effects of surgical treatment in thymoma with myasthenia gravis: our experience in 103 patients. J Surg Oncol 1992;50:43–6.

41. Wang L-S, Huang M-H, Lin T-S, et al. Malignant thymoma. Cancer 1992;70:443–50.

42. Elert O, Buchwald J, Wolf K. Epithelial thymus tumors—therapy and prognosis. Thorac Cardiovasc Surg 1988;36:109–13.

43. Kirschner PA. Reoperation for thymoma: report of 23 cases. Ann Thorac Surg 1990;49(4):550–4 [discussion: 555].

44. Zhu G, He S, Fu X, et al. Radiotherapy and prognostic factors for thymoma: a retrospective study of 175 patients. Int J Radiat Oncol Biol Phys 2004; 60(4):1113–9.

45. Levasseur P. Thymomas. In: Aisner J, Arriagada R, Green M, et al, editors. Comprehensive textbook of thoracic oncology. Baltimore (MD): Williams and Wilkins; 1996. p. 653–67.

46. Bernatz PE, Harrison EG, Clagett OT. Thymoma: a clinicopathologic study. J Thorac Cardiovasc Surg 1961;42(4):424–44.

47. Gamondès JP, Balawi A, Greenland T, et al. Seventeen years of surgical treatment of thymoma: factors influencing survival. Eur J Cardiothorac Surg 1991;5: 124–31.

48. Rubin M, Straus B, Allen L. Clinical disorders associated with thymic tumors. Arch Intern Med 1964;114:389.

49. Harvey AM. Some preliminary observations on the clinical course of myasthenia gravis before and after thymectomy. Bull N Y Acad Med 1948;24:505.

50. Fershtand JB, Shaw RR. Malignant tumor of thymus gland. Myasthenia gravis developing after removal. Ann Intern Med 1951;34:1025–35.

51. Nakagawa K, Asamura H, Matsuno Y, et al. Thymoma: a clinicopathologic study based on the new World Health Organization classification. J Thorac Cardiovasc Surg 2003;126(4):1134–40.

52. Deeb ME, Brinster CJ, Kucharzuk J, et al. Expanded indications for transcervical thymectomy in the management of anterior mediastinal masses. Ann Thorac Surg 2001;72:208–11.

53. Slater G, Papatestas AE, Kornfeld P, et al. Transcervical thymectomy for thymoma in myasthenia gravis. Am J Surg 1982;144:254–6.

54. Papatestas AE, Genkins G, Kornfeld P, et al. Effects of thymectomy in myasthenia gravis. Ann Surg 1987; 206:79–88.

55. Monden Y, Nakahara K, Iioka S, et al. Recurrence of thymoma: clinicopathological features, therapy and prognosis. Ann Thorac Surg 1985;39(2):165–9.

56. Cowen D, Richaud P, Mornex F, et al. Thymoma: results of a multicentric retrospective series of 149 non-metastatic irradiated patients and review of the literature. FNCLCC trialists. Federation Nationale des Centres de Lutte Contre le Cancer. Radiother Oncol 1995;34:9–16.

57. Pollack A, Komaki R, Cos JD, et al. Thymoma: treatment and prognosis. Int J Radiat Oncol Biol Phys 1992;23:1037–43.

58. Ogawa K, Uno T, Toita T, et al. Postoperative radiotherapy for patients with completely resected thymoma: a multi-institutional, retrospective review of 103 patients. Cancer 2002;94(5):1405–13.

59. Singhal S, Shrager JB, Rosenthal DI, et al. Comparison of stages I-II thymoma treated by complete resection with or without adjuvant radiation. Ann Thorac Surg 2003;76(5):1635–41 [discussion: 1641–32].

60. Mangi AA, Wright CD, Allan JS, et al. Adjuvant radiation therapy for stage II thymoma. Ann Thorac Surg 2002;74(4):1033–7.

61. Mangi AA, Wain JC, Donahue DM, et al. Adjuvant radiation of stage III thymoma: is it necessary? Ann Thorac Surg 2005;79(6):1834–9.

62. Korst RJ, Kansler AL, Christos PJ, et al. Adjuvant radiotherapy for thymic epithelial tumors: a systematic

review and meta-analysis. Ann Thorac Surg 2009;
87(5):1641–7.

63. Levine GD, Rosai J. Thymic hyperplasia and
neoplasia: a review of current concepts. Hum Pathol
1978;9(5):495–515.

64. Pescarmona E, Rendina EA, Venuta F, et al. The
prognostic implication of thymoma histologic subtyping: a study of 80 consecutive cases. Am J Clin
Pathol 1990;93:190–5.

65. Verley JM, Hollmann KH. Thymoma: a comparative
study of clinical stages, histologic features, and
survival in 200 cases. Cancer 1985;55(5):
1074–86.

66. Ruffini E, Mancuso M, Oliaro A, et al. Recurrence of
thymoma: analysis of clinicopathologic features,
treatment, and outcome. J Thorac Cardiovasc Surg
1997;113:55–63.

67. Masaoka A, Monden Y, Nakahara K, et al. Follow-up
study of thymomas with special reference to their
clinical stages. Cancer 1981;48:2485–92.

68. Pescarmona E, Rendina E, Venuta F, et al. Analysis
of prognostic factors and clinicopathological
staging of thymoma. Ann Thorac Surg 1990;50:
534–8.

69. Ströbel P, Bauer A, Puppe B, et al. Tumor recurrence
and survival in patients treated for thymomas and
thymic squamous cell carcinomas: a retrospective
analysis. J Clin Oncol 2004;22(8):1501–9.

70. Pan C-C, Wu H-P, Yang C-F, et al. The clinicopathological correlation of epithelial subtyping in thymoma:
a study of 112 consecutive cases. Hum Pathol 1994;
25:893–9.

71. Chalabreysse L, Roy P, Cordier J-F, et al. Correlation
of the WHO schema for the classification of thymic
epithelial neoplasms with prognosis. Am J Surg
Pathol 2002;26(12):1605–11.

72. Quintanilla-Martinez L, Wilkins EJ, Choi N, et al. Thymoma: histologic subclassification is an independent prognostic factor. Cancer 1994;74:606–17.

73. Dawson A, Ibrahim NBN, Gibbs AR. Observer variation in the histopathological classification of thymoma:
correlation with prognosis. J Clin Pathol 1994;47:
519–23.

74. Park MS, Chung KY, Kim KD, et al. Prognosis of
thymic epithelial tumors according to the new World
Health Organization histologic classification. Ann
Thorac Surg 2004;78(3):992–7 [discussion: 997–8].

75. Kondo K, Yoshizawa K, Tsuyuguchi M, et al. WHO
histologic classification is a prognostic indicator in
thymoma. Ann Thorac Surg 2004;77(4):1183–8.

76. Chen G, Marx A, Wen-Hu C, et al. New WHO histologic classification predicts prognosis of thymic
epithelial tumors: a clinicopathologic study of 200
thymoma cases from China. Cancer 2002;95(2):
420–9.

77. Regnard J-F, Zinzindohoue F, Magdeleinat P, et al.
Results of re-resection for recurrent thymomas.
Ann Thorac Surg 1997;64:1593–8.

78. Urgesi A, Monetti U, Rossi G, et al. Aggressive treatment of intrathoracic recurrences of thymoma. Radiother Oncol 1992;24:221–5.

79. Goldel N, Böning L, Fredrik A, et al. Chemotherapy
of invasive thymoma: a retrospective study of 22
cases. Cancer 1989;63:1493–500.

Minimally Invasive and Robotic-Assisted Thymus Resection

Karl K. Limmer, MD[a],*, Kemp H. Kernstine, MD, PhD[b]

KEYWORDS
- Thymoma • Minimally invasive • Robotics • Thymectomy
- Thoracoscopic • Myasthenia gravis

Thymectomy for thymoma has traditionally been performed through a transsternal approach because of the excellent exposure that that the median sternotomy provides. Minimally invasive alternatives, such as transcervical thymectomy, video-assisted thymectomy, and robotic thymectomy, have not been extensively evaluated for this disease process. It is uncertain which patients may benefit from minimally invasive approaches and data regarding the oncologic effectiveness of these techniques remains to be established. However, given the excellent capability of these techniques to perform a complete and extensive thymectomy, there does appear to be a role for minimally invasive thymectomy in the treatment of thymoma.

ANATOMY, HISTOLOGY, EMBRYOLOGY, AND FUNCTION OF THE THYMUS

Thymic tissue arises during the sixth week of gestation primarily from the third pharyngeal pouch with occasional contributions from the fourth pharyngeal pouch. The right and left lobes of the thymus develop separately; as each thymic lobe moves caudally the two lobes become connected but do not fuse. At full term, the thymus weighs approximately 15 g; it does not reach its greatest relative size until puberty, when it weighs 30 to 40 g on average. Throughout adulthood, the gland gradually decreases in size to approximately 5 to 25 g.[1]

In addition to the two classic lobes, thymic tissue may be found at ectopic sites throughout the mediastinum and cervical area. Ectopic foci may be present from the level of the thyroid gland to the diaphragm, an estimated 50% to 75% of thymic tissue is found in ectopic foci outside of the thymic capsule.[2,3] Primarily, the arterial blood supply originates from the internal mammary artery, additional blood is also supplied from the brachiocephalic, inferior thyroidal, and pericardiophrenic arteries. The venous drainage may accompany the arterial blood supply, but the most significant drainage is largely into the brachiocephalic vein.[4] There are occasional branches directly to the superior vena cava. The proximity of the thymus to other vital structures, such as the superior vena cava; brachiocephalic vein; and the phrenic, vagus, and recurrent laryngeal nerves, can make surgical dissection challenging. The complexity and variation of the thymic anatomy and the locations of ectopic foci are important when considering surgical indications and approaches to the thymus (**Fig. 1**).

DISEASES OF THE THYMUS
Indications for Thymectomy

The thymus functions in immunity and plays a central role in T-cell development. In postterm infants and into adulthood, removal of the thymus does not appear to alter immune function or capacity and it does not appear to be related to any identifiable clinical problem.[5] Surgical

[a] Department of Surgery, University of California San Diego School of Medicine, 200 West Arbor Drive, San Diego, CA 92103, USA
[b] Lung Cancer and Thoracic Oncology Program, City of Hope National Medical Center, 1500 East Duarte Road, Warsaw MOB, Suite 2001, Duarte, CA 91010, USA
* Corresponding author.
E-mail address: klimmer@ucsd.edu

Thorac Surg Clin 21 (2011) 69–83
doi:10.1016/j.thorsurg.2010.08.005
1547-4127/11/$ – see front matter

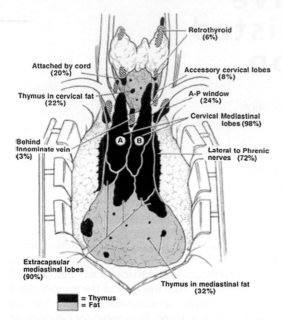

Fig. 1. Surgical anatomy of the thymus.

resection of the thymus is indicated in the presence of primary thymic malignancies, such as thymomas, thymic cysts, suspicious anterior mediastinal lesions, and myasthenia gravis (MG).[6,7]

Thymoma

Tumors arising from thymic epithelial cells are known as thymomas. Thymomas are rarely purely epithelial in nature, they are more commonly heterogeneous, consisting of thymic epithelial cells and lymphocytes in varying proportions. Tumors that originate from the lymphocytes are known as thymic lymphomas. Other tumor types include thymic carcinomas, carcinoid tumors, small cell cancer, and metastatic lesions. Thymomas are rare; the overall annual incidence is only 1.5 per 1,000,000; accounting for approximately 50% of all mediastinal masses.[8] At presentation, patients are usually in their sixties with no sex predilection; approximately one-half to one-third are symptomatic, usually with pressure-type discomfort, cough, dyspnea, or superior vena cava obstruction. Approximately one-third of patients with thymomas have myasthenia gravis. Additional paraneoplastic syndromes associated with thymomas include neuromuscular syndromes other than myasthenia gravis; hematologic syndromes, such as red cell aplasia; immunologic deficiency syndromes; collagen vascular and autoimmune disorders; dermatologic diseases; endocrine disorders; kidney dysfunction; hypertrophic osteoarthropathy; and malignancies, such

as lymphoma, Kaposi's sarcoma, and cancer of the lung and colon.[9] Approximately1 30% of patients with thymomas will develop an additional primary malignancy.[10,11]

Over the last several decades, several classification systems based upon various clinical[12–14] and histologic[15–17] features have been devised and used. The Masaoka stage is the most widely accepted clinical staging system at present (**Table 1**A). This system recognizes the importance of tumor capsular invasion, adjacent organ involvement, as well as locoregional and systemic metastases. The Masaoka stage can be assessed noninvasively with thoracic CT and it predicts the likelihood of tumor invasion and complete surgical resection. Because the ability to obtain a complete resection in thymoma is of the utmost importance, the Masaoka stage can be useful in determining which patients may benefit from neoadjuvant chemotherapy: those with more advanced Masaoka stage, lesions larger than 5 cm in greatest CT diameter, \those with imperceptible tissue planes between the mediastinal mass and adjacent mediastinal structures, or those thymomas that are less likely to be simply resected, such as those surrounding or involving the great vessels.

The World Health Organization (WHO) classification[18] is based upon cytologic differences between normal thymic epithelial cells and neoplastic cells (**Table 1**B). The system recognizes 6 types of thymic tumors, including thymic carcinoma, and classifies them into distinct groups. One important aspect of the WHO system is the ability to predict long-term outcomes on the basis of WHO type. In a meta-analysis of thymoma case series, the WHO type has been shown to be an independent predictor of disease-specific survival.[19] However, the clinical utility of this

Table 1A Masaoka stage	
Stage	**Definition**
I	Macroscopically completely encapsulated and microscopically no capsular invasion
II	Macroscopic invasion into surrounding fatty tissue of mediastinal pleura or microscopic invasion into capsule
III	Macroscopic invasion into neighboring organs (ie, pericardium great vessels or lung)
IVa	Pleural or pericardial dissemination
IVb	Hematogenous or lymphogenous metastasis

Table 1B
The new World Health Organization histologic classification of thymic epithelial tumors

Type	Histologic Description
A	Medullary thymoma
AB	Mixed thymoma
B1	Predominantly conical thymoma
B2	Cortical thymoma
B3	Well-differentiated thymic carcinoma
C	Thymic carcinoma

staging system may be limited in the initial evaluation of patients because the assignment of the WHO type requires that patients undergo a biopsy procedure to make a histologic diagnosis. Many surgeons would prefer to use the Masaoka stage to determine if the mass is likely to be resectable and would not routinely perform a biopsy for those tumors that appear to be resectable. In these cases, the WHO type would be assigned only after the decision to operate has been made and the tumor has been resected.

Evaluation of a patient with an anterior mediastinal mass suspicious for thymoma is directed toward determining if the mass is resectable. Other sources of anterior mediastinal mass should be considered and ruled out. The determination of normal serum lactate dehydrogenase (LDH) is used to assess for the presence of lymphoma. Elevation of serum alpha-fetoprotein or beta-HCG (human chorionic gonadotropin) indicate a high likelihood for a malignant germ cell tumor.

A high-quality thoracic CT scan should be performed to determine the potential for complete resection. The scan will determine the size of the thymic mass, evaluate the mass for signs of local invasion, and rule out metastatic disease. Findings on CT that predict invasion include: tumor size greater than 5 cm, tumors abutting the flat plane of the pericardium and lung for a significant distance, as well as the more obvious signs of tumor invagination into the interstices of the great vessels or perhaps completely surrounding them. Tumors that are small and are surrounded by normal tissue planes are most likely to be completely resectable; the size of the thymoma is inversely related to the likelihood of complete R0 resection. Those patients who are symptomatic at the time of presentation are more likely to have tumor invasion.[20]

When the WHO tumor type is known preoperatively, this information may be used to determine which patients are appropriate for minimally invasive thymectomy. In 2002, Okumura and colleagues[21] correlated the WHO classification to the Masaoka stage and determined the likelihood of tumor invasion for each WHO type (**Table 2**). In addition to demonstrating an association between WHO tumor types and Masoka stage, this study showed that WHO class could be useful in determining the likelihood of tumor invasion. As seen in **Table 2**, Type A tumors are more likely Masaoka stage I and are unlikely to invade with only 10% to 45% demonstrating invasion of the capsule or beyond; whereas, type AB, B1, B2, and B3 are more likely associated with advanced stage and invasion, 35% to 70% for AB, B1, and B2 and up to 85% for B3. The WHO tumor type does not appear to offer any management direction for masses on preoperative imaging that are less than 5 cm and have clear margins and fat around them. Those patients are highly likely to achieve an R0 resection. However, for the larger lesions and those with indistinct planes, preoperative diagnosis and subtype determination may assist in determining prognosis and treatment planning. Thus, the WHO stage is not known until the surgery has been performed and may be of little clinical relevance in determining potential resectability.

In the authors' practice, they do not routinely biopsy well-circumscribed anterior mediastinal

Table 2
Likelihood of tumor invasion based upon WHO tumor type

| Variable | WHO Tumor Type | | | | | |
	A	AB	B1	B2	B3	Total
Number of patients	18	77	55	97	26	273
Invasive tumors (%) a	2 (11.1)	32 (41.6)	26 (47.3)	67 (69.1)	22 (84.6)	149
GV involved (%) b	0 (0)	3 (3.9)	4 (7.3)	17 (17.5)	5 (19.2)	29

Abbreviations: GV, great vessels; WHO, World Health Organization.
Data from Olumura M, Ohta M, and Tateyama H, et al. The World Health Organization histologic classification system rejects the oncologic behavior of thymoma: a clinical study of 273 patients. Cancer 2002;94:624–32.

masses that appear consistent with thymoma. Asymptomatic patients with this finding are thought to have a low likelihood of invasion and are therefore offered surgical resection. The authors reserve biopsy for patients with large tumors, tumors that are not clearly thymomas, or tumors that appear to be invasive on CT. The practice of selective biopsies is based upon the theoretical risk that a biopsy may disturb the capsule and spread malignant cells. Percutaneous fine-needle biopsy of an anterior mediastinal lesion with a 20-gauge needle establishes a definitive diagnosis in 84% of cases.[22] If this does not provide a diagnosis, the authors perform an anterior mediastinotomy (Chamberlin procedure) with incisional biopsy to make the diagnosis. Patients with suspicion of invasion and advanced histologic type are less likely to have a complete surgical resection[21] and are offered induction chemotherapy or chemoradiotherapy before surgery. It has been demonstrated that this approach for advanced Masaoka Stage III thymomas offers improved disease-free and overall survival as compared with chemoradiotherapy following resection.[23]

The goal of surgical resection is the complete resection of the thymic mass with en bloc resection of adjacent nonvital structures and metastatic deposits. In addition to the complete resection of the entire thymus, it is important to maintain the capsule surrounding the tumor, avoiding tumor spillage. Nonvital structures that are involved with the thymic mass, such as the pericardium, pleura, and pulmonary parenchyma, should be

resected. Consideration can be given to resecting one of the phrenic nerves in patients who are non-myasthenic if this maneuver will result in an R0 resection. If there is bilateral phrenic nerve involvement, then an R0 resection cannot be obtained and a reductive surgery is performed. The brachiocephalic vein and possibly the superior vena cava may also be resected and may be reconstructed with a spiral vein or prosthetic interposition graft. Areas where surgical margins are close should be marked with metallic clips and the specimen should be oriented for pathology.

Surgical resection does not improve survival or quality of life in all patients; however, numerous case series have demonstrated that the main factor associated with long-term survival in thymoma is the completeness of resection.[21,24-28] These studies show significant survival advantage at 5 and 10 years in those patients undergoing complete R0 resections (**Table 3**).[29] Rea and colleagues[25] found no survival difference in groups of subjects undergoing debulking surgery versus diagnostic biopsy alone. This finding calls into question the role for debulking surgery in thymoma; however, a later study providing 35-year follow-up of 317 subjects surgically treated for thymoma found that only 10 of 22 subjects (45%) who were treated with incomplete resection had clinically significant relapse of the disease at follow-up.[30] The low recurrence rate in this group of subjects provides some evidence that continued surgical debulking may have a role in the treatment of advanced thymoma.

Table 3
Thymoma survival according to extent of resection

| | Survival According to Extent of Resection | | | | | | |
	Rea	Zhu	Nakagawa	Regnard	Kim	Okum	Margaritora
Patients	132	175	130	307	108	273	317
Complete resection	81.8%	72.0%	95.0%	84.7%	81.5%	94.5%	93.1%
5-y SR	82.5%	88.4%	96.0%	—	81.5%	94.5%	92%
10-y SR	71.0%	—	94.0%	76.0%	85.0%	95.0%	87.4%
20-y SR	—	—	—	—	—	—	77.0%
Incomplete resection	9.1%	13.7%	5.0%	9.8%	18.5%	3.3%	6.9%
5-y SR	16.0%	43.2%	33.0%	—	55.0%	—	73.0%
10-y SR	9.0%	—	33.0%	28.0%	35.0%	60.0%	32.0%
20-y SR	—	—	—	—	—	—	21.0%
Biopsy/gross disease	9.1%	14.4%	—	5.5%	—	1.6%	—
5-y SR	33.0%	73.5%	—	—	—	—	—

Abbreviation: SR, survival rate.
Significant Data from Tomaszek S, Wigle DA, Keshavjee S, et al. Thymomas: review of current clinical practice. Ann Thorac Surg 2009;87:1973–80.

Myasthenia Gravis

Thymomas are frequently associated with para-neoplastic disorders, the most common being myasthenia gravis. MG is an autoimmune disorder caused by autoimmunity against the acetylcholine receptor (AChR). The disease prevalence is estimated to be 1 in 5000 to 1 in 10,000.[31] The disease is characterized by skeletal muscle fatigue and weakness resulting from competitive inhibition of the receptor and complement-mediated destruction of the AChR.[32-34] The muscular fatigue is exacerbated by repetitive movements and is alleviated by rest. The role of the thymus in myasthenia gravis was first proposed by Oppenheim, a German neurologist who discovered a thymic tumor at autopsy in a patient with myasthenia gravis.[35] The presence of a thymoma is not required to produce MG; however, more severe disease is associated with the presence of thymoma.[36] Myasthenia gravis is more prevalent in the more advanced WHO thymoma tissue type with 14% found in type A and nearly 50% found in B3.

The diagnosis of MG is established by provocative testing of the neuromuscular junction (NMJ) pharmacologically or via electromyography (EMG).[37] The most sensitive diagnostic test being EMG with repetitive nerve stimulation. Repetitive nerve stimulation demonstrates a decreased excitatory postsynaptic potential in patients who are myasthenic as acetylcholine is depleted in the NMJ.[38,39] Pharmacologic testing is performed with edrophonium,[37] a short-acting acetylcholinesterase inhibitor that increases the concentration of acetylcholine at the neuromuscular junction. With administration of edrophonium, patients with MG may clinically improve. This test is 97% sensitive for MG.[39] Additionally, antibody testing for acetylcholine receptor antibody is highly disease specific for MG, although antibody levels do not correlate with disease severity.[40] Disease severity and classification have been formally addressed by the Myasthenia Gravis Foundation of America.[41,42]

Medical management of MG is initiated with acetylcholinesterase inhibitors, such as neostigmine and pyridostigmine; however, prolonged use of these agents may potentially exacerbate the damaging effects of MG.[43] Long-term corticosteroids may also be used to suppress the effects of MG. Initiation of steroids may initially worsen the symptoms of MG, but improvement is typically seen after 3 to 6 weeks of treatment. Immunosuppressive regimens are also useful to modulate the disease. Azathioprine or cyclosporine may be added in patients who experience only partial relief with steroids or who are not able to tolerate the side effects of steroids. Further treatment with intravenous immunoglobulin or plasmapheresis may also be of benefit in select patients.

The role of thymectomy in the treatment of nonthymomatous myasthenia gravis remains controversial. Thymectomy has provided cure in some, but not all, patients with myasthenia gravis.[44-48] Some experts advocate for thymectomy early in the disease course, although, others reserve thymectomy for those patients who are failing medical management. Although indications and approaches to thymectomy remain controversial, thymectomy in patients with MG has become the standard of care. When surgical intervention is being considered, the entire clinical picture must be assessed. Factors that favor surgical intervention include increased disease severity, disease duration, patient age, and overall fitness for surgery. Thymoma will be present in 10% to 15% of patients with MG and is an indication for resection. In patients with MG, CT has a false negative rate for thymoma of approximately 10%.[49] Thymectomy, especially when performed early in the disease course, has been shown to be associated with increased rates of disease remission.[36] Because of the presence of ectopic thymic tissue in the perithymic mediastinal fat and other mediastinal locations, the extent of thymectomy may be associated with superior rates of remission from myasthenia gravis,[50] as high as 86% at 10 years. There is currently a multicenter phase III clinical trial underway to define the role of thymectomy in MG.[51]

Thymic Cysts

Anterior mediastinal cystic masses originating from the thymus are an infrequent finding, representing less than 5% of cystic masses of the mediastinum.[52] Typically, these masses are asymptomatic, but they may also be associated with pain or other symptoms related to mass effect of the cysts. On diagnostic ultrasonography, the lesions are typically identified as simple cystic lesions. CT will also reveal a simple mass; multiloculated lesions should raise the suspicion of thymoma.

Thymic cysts may be derived from congenital origins or acquired as a result of involutional changes of the gland.[52] In addition, thymic cysts may also be present in the anterior cervical neck.

Diagnosis and treatment of thymic cysts is uncertain. Percutaneous fine-needle aspiration or mediastinoscopy with needle aspiration of the cyst may not be useful in the diagnosis or treatment of these lesions.[53] Lesions causing significant symptoms or those that are suspicious for thymoma should be surgically removed.

HISTORY OF SURGICAL TREATMENT

Surgery of the thymus has evolved over the last century. The first report of a successful thymectomy was made in 1911 by Ferdinand Sauerbruch, who performed a cervical thymectomy on a patient with MG.[54] Following this initial report, it was not until 1936 that Alfred Blalock described the transsternal thymectomy.[55] He later followed up his initial report with a case series of 20 myasthenic subjects who were successfully treated with surgery.[56] Sternotomy is regarded by many as the gold standard surgical approach to the thymus. Advantages of the sternotomy include excellent visualization of the thymus and surrounding structures as well as the ability to extend the incision in order to resect and reconstruct all involved structures in cases of advanced thymic pathology.[29] In addition, many surgeons believe that open approach provides the most oncologically sound operation and eliminates the risk of drop metastasis resulting from minimally invasive approaches. In the treatment of MG, the sternotomy allows for a very thorough exploration of the mediastinum.[50]

Transcervical thymectomy, as first described at the beginning of the twentieth century, can be considered the first minimally invasive approach to thymectomy. This technique involves a supracervical incision with dissection in a retrosternal plane to remove thymic tissue. In the late 1960s, Kark reported on a series of transcervical thymectomies in MG.[57] In this comparative study, there were fewer postoperative complications in the transcervical group compared with the transsternal cases. The decreased rate of complications led to the greater acceptance of surgical intervention and operations for patients with MG earlier in the disease course. Later, the addition of the Cooper retractor improved the transcervical exposure by elevating the sternum.[58] Further improvement was made by de Perrot and colleagues[59] using a video endoscope to directly visualize the deeper recesses within the mediastinum.

Traditionally, transcervical thymectomy was reserved for patients who were nonthymomatous myasthenic. This technique produced results that are equivalent to transsternal resection.[60,61] In 2001, Deeb and colleagues[7] published one of the first case series that included thymomas up to 5 cm in size as long as no sign of invasion was found on CT.

With the advancement of endoscopic equipment and techniques, video-assisted thoracic surgery (VATS) was used to resect the thymus.[62] At that time, the authors of this first case report were criticized for incompletely treating the patient. Later, continued interest in VATS led to the first successful case series of the VATS technique in MG[63,64] and thymoma.[65]

Further advancement of surgical technology led to the development and approval of the da Vinci (Intuitive Surgical, Sunnyvale, CA, USA) robotic surgical system. The first robotic procedure performed was a chole-cystectomy in 1998. As further experience was obtained with the surgical robot, it became clear that one of the strengths of the technology was the improved ability to perform complex surgical procedures in small anatomic spaces. The fact that the mediastinum is an area where the surgical robot may facilitate precise surgery led Yoskino to perform the first robotic thymectomy in 2001 in a 74-year-old man with a 3.5 cm thymoma.[66] Since that time, the number of robotic thymectomies has continued to increase. In 2009, nearly 400 thymectomies were performed with the da Vinci surgical system (**Fig. 2**).

PREOPERATIVE PREPARATION

Preoperative preparation of patients undergoing thymectomy for any reason should be thorough. Standard preoperative workup, including basic laboratories, electrocardiogram, and chest radiographs, should be performed. A blood gas performed on room air is useful in determining if patients will be capable of tolerating the single lung ventilation that is required for VATS or robot-assisted thymectomy. If there is any concern that a patient's pulmonary disease may be limiting, pulmonary function testing should be performed. Evaluation of the chest CT will further aid in preoperative planning.

In patients with MG, additional measures must be taken to optimize them for surgery by maximizing neuromuscular transmission, decreasing circulating antibody levels, and suppressing the

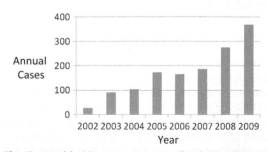

Fig. 2. Worldwide annual cases of robotic thymectomy. (*Data from* Intuitive Surgical, Inc, Sunnyvale, CA; *Obtained from* Dr Jens Ruckert and Dr Mahmoud Ismail, Charite Hospital, Berlin, Germany; with permission.)

immune response. In the weeks leading up to surgery, anticholinesterase inhibitors should be minimized to reduce the potential chances for postoperative bronchorrhea or rhinorrhea. The reduction in acetylcholinesterase inhibitors should be done while maintaining symptomatic control. On the morning of surgery, a one-half dose of acetylcholinesterase inhibitors is given to patients with mild symptoms. Patients who are experiencing significant symptoms should receive a full dose on the morning of surgery. In an effort to minimize the complications of steroids, those patients who are maintained with steroids should have their dose titrated down to the lowest possible level that still maintains an acceptable level of symptomatic relief. Plasmapheresis for patients whose symptoms are uncontrolled by medications should be continued. In addition, perioperative plasmapheresis may allow for successful weaning of steroids and may reduce the risk of perioperative respiratory complications.[67–69]

The anesthetic plan should be discussed with the anesthesiologist before surgery. The stress of the surgery may precipitate complications in patients who are myasthenic. Long-standing muscular fatigue increases the likelihood that patients with MG will require additional ventilatory support following the case. Depolarizing neuromuscular junction blockers, such as succinylcholine, are less likely to be effective in these patients and more likely to result in ventilatory support after surgery. Preoperative plasmapheresis may also complicate anesthesia by removing plasma cholinesterases that are responsible for metabolizing nondepolarizing agents, such as atracurium.

OPERATIVE TECHNIQUES
Transcervical and Video-Assisted Transcervical Approaches

Transcervical thymectomy proceeds by placing the patient in the supine position with a bean bag under the thorax. Anesthesia is obtained and a single lumen endotracheal tube is placed and taped to the side of the patient. The positioning of the endotracheal tube is important; a significant portion of the operation will be performed from the head of the bed with the surgeon in the seated position peering over the patient's head. The patient's neck is fully extended but is supported and is not allowed to hang above the bed. In addition to the neck, the chest is also prepared and draped for surgery in case a median sternotomy is required to completely remove a thymoma or to control bleeding.

A mini-collar incision is made in a skin crease 2 fingerbreadths above the sternal notch. A subplatysmal flap is then developed inferiorly. Dissection is carried down until the strap muscles are identified. The strap muscles are incised longitudinally and then retracted laterally. The origins of the sternocleidomastoid muscle are divided from the clavicles bilaterally to provide additional exposure of the mediastinum. The superior poles of the thymus are identified just deep to the sternocleidomastoid and are then ligated and divided with silk ligatures. The sutures are not cut but are left as long tags from the thymus to provide gentle caudle traction that aids in dissection and exposure (**Fig. 3**A). Dissection continues inferiorly and posteriorly until the thymic poles coalesce to form the single thymic body at the level of the innominate vein. Blunt dissection of the posterior sternal table with a finger or other blunt instrument develops the anterior thymic plane (see **Fig. 3**B). Once an adequate surface of the sternum has been cleared of thymic tissue, the Cooper retractor is placed directly beneath the sternum. The retractor is tightened to slightly elevate the thorax from the operative field (see **Fig. 3**C). The additional exposure that is provided by elevating the sternum allows for the anterior dissection of the thymus to be completed. The use of the video endoscope at this point may also aid in the anterior dissection by providing additional light and a magnified image on the video monitor (see **Fig. 3**D). The video endoscope has the additional benefit of allowing more than one surgeon to have optimal visualization of the operative field. The posterior dissection is completed by pulling on the traction sutures to expose the posterior surface of the thymus. The venous drainage of the thymus into the brachiocephalic vein is identified posteriorly and is ligated with clips and divided. Laterally, the arterial blood supply enters from the internal mammary artery. These branches are also clipped and divided. If visualization is difficult, reducing the tidal volumes and respiratory rate may help to facilitate the necessary exposure. Additional blunt dissection of the inferior poles should free the thymus from the pericardium and pleura. A complete evaluation of the mediastinum is performed to evaluate for any remaining or ectopic thymic tissue.

VATS Thymectomy

VATS thymectomy can be performed through the left or right chest. The right side is favored by many because of the increased space in the right chest as well as the improved access and visibility of the venous structures.

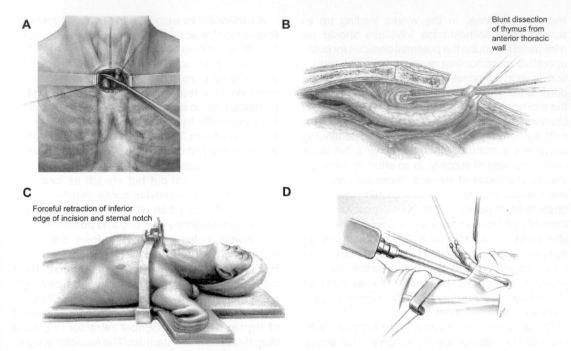

Fig. 3. Transcervical thymectomy (A–D). (Reprinted from de Perrot M, Keshavjee S. Video-assisted transcervical thymectomy. Operat Tech Thorac Cardiovasc Surg 2005;10(3):220–30; and Meyers BF. Transcervical thymectomy. Operat Tech Thorac Cardiovasc Surg 2001;6(4):201–8; with permission.)

Single-lung ventilation is required. The patient is placed in the left-lateral decubitus position with a roll placed under the axilla. The operative focus is superior and anterior mediastinum, thus the ports are placed relatively anteriorly and superiorly (Fig. 4A). It should be kept in mind that the operative field is somewhat remote from the port sites and that the final relationships of the instruments should be accounted for when choosing port sites to optimize the function of each of the ports. Generally, 4 ports are placed: 1 for the video scope, 2 for the dissecting instruments, and 1 for retraction, as necessary.

Once the ports have been placed, CO2 is insufflated to improve visualization by distention of the mediastinum to the left, compression of the lung away from the operative field, and clearing the field of cautery smoke. The right phrenic nerve is identified and preserved. The mediastinal pleura are incised longitudinally and blunt dissection of the mediastinum identifies the inferior pole of the thymus. Dissection continues in a plane posterior to the thymus; attachments of the thymus to the sternum may be left in place initially. Venous branches draining into the brachiocephalic vein and superior vena cave are identified, clipped, and divided. The thymus is placed on gentle traction and the dissection is performed over the pericardium toward the contralateral inferior thymic pole (see Fig. 4B). The anterior attachments of the thymus are taken down and the superior pole is identified. The blood supply to the thymus is clipped and divided. The thymus is placed into an endoscopic retrieval bag and is removed from one of the port sites.

Robotic Thymectomy

Robotic thymectomy is gaining acceptance and has been performed by the isolated left- or right-sided approach as well as with a bilateral approach. In general, the authors find that the right-sided approach is advantageous. The absence of the heart on the right side creates additional space and allows for greater visualization and access to the contralateral side.[70] In addition, the presence of the vena cava and brachiocephalic veins clearly delineates the surgical anatomy and allows for precise dissection of thymic tissue. In situations where the bulk of the thymus or thymic mass predominates on the left side, a primarily left-sided approach is used because of the improved visualization of the AP window and possibly decreased risk of phrenic nerve injury.[71] More recently in our series, we tend to prepare the patient for a bilateral approach to ensure complete removal of all thymic tissue.

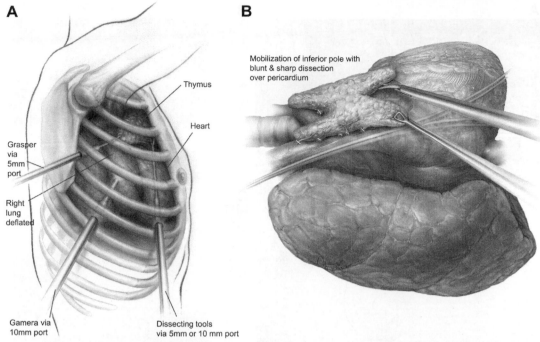

A

Thymus

Heart

Grasper
via
5mm
port

Right
lung
deflated

Gamera via
10mm port

Dissecting tools
via 5mm or 10 mm port

B

Mobilization of inferior pole with
blunt & sharp dissection
over pericardium

Fig. 4. VATS. (*Reprinted from* Hazelrigg SR. Thoracoscopic or video-assisted (VATS) thymectomy. Operat Tech Thorac Cardiovasc Surg 2004;9(2):184–92; with permission.)

Patient positioning is critical for successful robotic thymectomy. Great care should be taken to properly position patients before engaging the robot. Single-lung ventilation is usually required, but not absolutely necessary. The patient is positioned in a modified supine position with the right side elevated 30° from horizontal (or left side if the left approach is being used) with the well-padded right arm dropped below the level of the operating table to provide exposure to the right axilla (**Fig. 5**A). This position uses gravity to assist in retraction of the hilum and lung away from the anterior mediastinum. Next, the patient's neck is extended and the head is positioned gently to the opposite side. With an indelible pen and using the chest CT as a guide, we mark out the presumed location of the thymus onto the anterior chest wall and then place marks for a possible emergent median sternotomy or transcervical neck incision to gain access for bleeding control or assist in removal of insufficiently visualized areas should problems occur (see **Fig. 5**B). Once the area of the thymus is marked, a position for the camera port is chosen that is opposite to and at a sufficient distance from the mark to permit adequate insertion and range of the scope. During this port placement, it must be kept in mind that the area that will require visualization during thymectomy is large and the camera must be able to access all areas of the mediastinum.

Once the site for the camera is chosen, a triangle is drawn toward the operative site with the port at the apex. This triangle demonstrates the site lines and working range of the camera; all additional ports should be kept outside of the lines to ensure unobstructed view and function of the video port and robotic arms (see **Fig. 5**C).

Exposure is facilitated by insufflation with CO_2 and by the use of paddle retractors on the anterior mediastinal structures. If it is not possible to completely expose the contralateral mediastinum with retraction alone, additional measures can be taken to improve access. Positive end-expiratory pressure can be added to the contralateral lung or CO_2 insufflation pressure can be decreased to move the mediastinal structures closer to the robotic ports. Additionally, the robotic ports may be repositioned to a different rib interspace through the same skin incision. If these measures do not allow adequate access to the intended operative site, approaching the mass from the contralateral side must be considered.

Once a total of 4 ports are placed and using a 0°scope, the procedure begins by identifying the phrenic nerve on the right side in the same fashion as the VATS approach. A pericardial plane is developed and once sufficient pericardium is cleared, gentle retraction of the heart with the endoscopic paddle retractor will provide additional exposure, especially to the left-sided

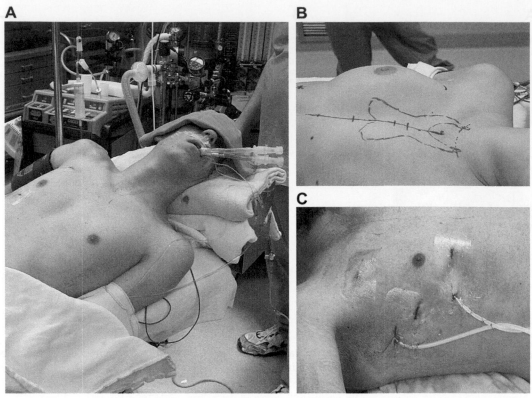

Fig. 5. Patient position with both arms tucked and patient rotated 30° from horizontal (*A*). Markings of thymic tissue and alternative transcervical and transsternal incisions (*B*). Final port and drain placement following successful right-sided robot-assisted thymectomy (*C*).

structures, such as the phrenic nerve. Different than the VATS approach, the sternal attachments of the thymus are left in place until the pericardial plane is fully developed and the inferior dissection is complete. By doing so, it prevents the thymic tissue from falling into the areas of dissection, obstructing the view, and minimizes any retraction or grasping of the specimen until it is ready to be placed into the endoscopic retrieval bag for retrieval at the end of the case. Dissection is performed to the brachiocephalic vein where the left phrenic nerve is identified in the left phrenopericardial angle. Once the phrenic nerve is identified, dissection continues until the entire circumference of the brachiocephalic vein is cleared and all mediastinal tissue is removed from the anterolateral aspects of the great vessels. The dissection is completed superiorly by identifying and removing all cervical tissue. All mediastinal tissue is removed via an endoscopic retrieval bag.

SUMMARY

The primary surgical objective in the treatment of thymoma is the complete resection of the tumor, including any nonvital involved structures.

Although it is not possible to safely remove all thymomas via a minimally invasive approach, it can no longer be stated that the presence of thymoma is a contraindication to minimally invasive thymectomy.

Thymectomy through median sternotomy was the preferred approach for many years. The acceptance of transcervical thymectomy increased with the addition of the sternal retractor that improved access to and visualization of the mediastinum. Numerous case series of transcervical thymectomy have been published primarily for the treatment of MG. However, the presence of thymoma has been considered a contraindication to transcervical thymectomy. As a result, the majority of thymomas removed through the transcervical approach were either small or were found incidentally following thymectomy for MG. The removal of clearly noninvasive, small (<4 cm) thymomas, has been advocated for by Deeb in his series of 28 attempted thymoma resections from this approach.[7] In total, 23 of 28 subjects underwent successful transsternal resection. Five required additional incisions, including 3 median sternotomies, 1 upper sternal splitting, and 1 left VATS. Follow-up ranged from 3 to 96 months and no tumor recurrence was noted. Based on this report, it appears that transcervical thymectomy in small noninvasive tumors is suitable. Additional long-term follow-up in a large group of subjects will be needed to determine applicability.

VATS thymectomy has been gaining popularity in the treatment of MG. When compared with transsternal thymectomy in MG, VATS thymectomy has been shown to be associated with decreased intraoperative blood loss,[72–74] decreased hospital stay,[72,75,76] and decreased pain[77] while producing similar long-term outcomes.[72–74,76,78]

In regards to robotic thymectomy, there have been a number of groups reporting results for this procedure in MG (**Table 4**).[70,71,79–85] Operative times were between 120 to 175 minutes, and hospital stays were between 2 to 4 days. No mortalities were reported; bleeding was the most common complication. There was 1 report of phrenic nerve injury and there were 8 reported conversions. Half of the investigators reported a predominantly right-sided approach; whereas, the other half reported a predominantly left-sided approach.

The literature is less robust for minimally invasive thymoma resection. There are a few case series, but the numbers are low and the follow-up is short term.[62,65,86–91] At least one attempt has been made to clearly define the criteria with which patients may be selected for a minimally invasive thymoma resection.[90] Without conversion, VATS thymectomy for thymoma was successfully performed in 44 subjects: 27 subjects with stage I tumors and 17 subjects with stage II tumors. The investigators did not offer VATS thymoma resection to any subjects who demonstrated significant pain, hoarseness, signs of vena caval obstruction, or diaphragm dysfunction. The CT finding of normal mediastinal fat plane preservation was considered a requisite feature

for VATS approach. The mean tumor size was 7.1 cm for stage I tumors and 8.5 cm for stage II; one patient had a tumor that was 18 cm in greatest dimension. The investigators of this study also compared the results of 11 minimally invasive stage II thymoma resections to a matched group of subjects undergoing transsternal resections.[65] The VATS group had a significantly less blood loss and there was no difference in operative time, duration of chest tube drainage, or hospital stay. There were no recurrences in either group at a mean follow-up of 33.9±19.7 months. Unfortunately, it is not clear how the decision of VATS or transsternal resection was made and the follow-up is not long enough to assess the outcome from either surgical technique in a disease that is more likely to recur beyond 5 to 10 years.

The enthusiasm for minimally invasive approaches must be tempered by the realities of what can be performed safely with these approaches. It does not appear that large tumor size necessarily prohibits a minimally invasive approach. However, there are limitations. The transcervical approach may not safely accommodate a large mass passing through the cervical incision or the thoracic inlet. Minimally invasive approaches should not be attempted in tumors that are severely adherent or invasive into vital structures. With the current robotic and minimally invasive technology, if reconstruction of the brachiocephalic vein or superior vena cave is required, these approaches are not suitable.

The widespread adoption of robotic thymectomy will be significantly improved when clearly defined surgical indications are established. With the majority of published experience in robotic thymectomy consisting of small case series with little long-term follow-up, it is difficult to draw conclusions about appropriate indications and patient selection. The various criteria that Cheng[90]

Table 4
Summary of robotic thymectomy case series

Author	Augustin	Rea	Savitt	Ruckert	Fleck	Castle	Goldstein	Total
Patients (n)	22	33	15	106	18	26	26	242
Approach	NR	Left	Right	Left	Left side	Right	Right	NA
Conversion	1	0	0	1	1	1	4	8
OR time (min)	134 (54–314)	120	96 (62–132)	NR	175 ± 6	90	127 ± 35	NA
Postoperative stay (d)	NR	2.6 (2–14)	2	NR	4 ± 1.8 d	1.6	2 (1–4)	NA

Abbreviations: NA, not applicable; NR, not reported; OR, operating room.

has outlined for selecting patients (asymptomatic patients with radiologic evidence of noninvasive Masaoka stage I or II tumors) appear to lead to a reasonable level of technical success. The future work in minimally invasive and robotic mediastinal surgery should not only be directed at clarifying surgical indications and limitation, but also identifying which patients may receive additional benefit from minimally invasive surgical techniques. For instance, patients with MG are often maintained on large doses of steroids, which can adversely affect wound healing. How much prednisone is too much to perform median sternotomy when a minimally invasive approach may provide an equivalent result with decreased potential for major wound complications? Are the smaller incisions and decreased pain worth the potential difference in outcomes? If there is no tumor invasion, is the risk of violating and seeding the pleura too great? If patients have suspected lung or pleural involvement, is a VATS or robotic approach preferred over sternotomy to remove the involved lung parenchyma? It remains to be seen if the theoretical oncologic benefits produce meaningful differences in the results between traditional and minimally invasive thymectomy. As further technological advances continue to expand the possibilities for minimally invasive thymectomy, additional randomized trials with long-term follow-up will be needed to clearly define the appropriate role of this technology in thymectomy.

REFERENCES

1. Shields TW. The thymus. In: Shields TW, editor. General thoracic surgery. 6th edition. Philadelphia: Lippincott Williams & Wilkins; 2005. p. 2347–56.
2. Fukai I, Funato Y, Mizuno T, et al. Distribution of thymic tissue in the mediastinal adipose tissue. J Thorac Cardiovasc Surg 1991;101:1099–102.
3. Tabatabaie SA, Hashemi SM, Sanei B, et al. The frequency of ectopic thymic tissue in the necks of patients without any thymic disease. Med Sci Monit 2007;13:CR283–5.
4. Di Marino V, Argeme M, Brunet C, et al. Macroscopic study of the adult thymus. Surg Radiol Anat 1987; 9(1):51–62.
5. Adner MM, Ise C, Schwab R, et al. Immunologic studies of thymectomized and nonthymectomized patients with myasthenia gravis. Ann N Y Acad Sci 1966;135(1):536–54.
6. Jaretzki A III. Thymectomy for myasthenia gravis: analysis of controversies - patient management. Neurologist 2003;9:77–92.
7. Deeb ME, Brister OJ, Kucharzuk J, et al. Expanded indications for transcervical thymectomy in the

8. Engels EA, Pfeiffer RM. Malignant thymoma in the United States: demographic patterns in incidence and associations with subsequent malignancies. Int J Cancer 2003;105(4):546–51.
9. Marchessky AM, Kaneko M. Surgical pathology of the mediastinum. New York: Raven Press; 1992.
10. Welsh JS, Wilkins KB, Green R, et al. Association between thymoma and second neoplasms. JAMA 2000;283(9):1142–3.
11. Welsh JS, Thurman SA, Howard SP. Thymoma and multiple malignancies: a case of five synchronous neoplasms and literature review. Clin Med Res 2003;1(3):227–32.
12. Masaoka A, Monden Y, Nakahara K, et al. Follow-up study of thymomas with special reference to their clinical stages. Cancer 1981;48:2485–92.
13. Koga K, Matsuno Y, Noguchi M, et al. A review of 79 thymomas: modification of staging system and reappraisal of conventional division into invasive and non-invasive thymoma. Pathol Int 1994;44:359–67.
14. Yamakawa Y, Masaoka A, Hashimoto T, et al. A tentative tumor-node-metastasis classification of thymoma. Cancer 1991;68:1984–7.
15. Rosai J, Sobin L, World Health Organization. Histological typing of tumours of the thymus. In: World Health Organization, editor. International histological classification of tumours. Heidelberg (Germany): Springer; 1999. p. 1–16.
16. Levine GD, Rosai J. Thymic hyperplasia and neoplasia: a review of current concepts. Hum Pathol 1978;9:495–515.
17. Marino M, Muller-Hermelink H. Thymoma and thymic carcinoma: Relation of thymoma epithelial cells to the cortical and medullary differentiation of the thymus. Virchows Arch A Pathol Anat Histopathol 1985;407:119–49.
18. Múller-Hermelink HK, Ströbel P, Zettl A, et al. Combined thymic epithelial tumours. In: Travis WD, Brambilla E, Múller-Hermelink HK, et al, editors. Pathology and genetics of tumours of the lung, pleura, thymus and heart (WHO classification of tumours series). Lyon (France): IARC Press; 2004. p. 196–8.
19. Detterbeck FC. Clinical value of the WHO classification system of thymoma. Ann Thorac Surg 2006;81: 2328–34.
20. Wright CD, Wain JC, Wong DR, et al. Predictors of recurrence in thymic tumors: importance of invasion, World Health Organization histology, and size. J Thorac Cardiovasc Surg 2005;130(5):1413–21.
21. Okumura M, Ohta M, Tateyama H, et al. The World Health Organization histologic classification system reflects the oncologic behavior of thymoma: a clinical study of 273 patients. Cancer 2002;94: 624–32.

22. Assaad MW, Pantanowitz L, Otis CN. Diagnostic accuracy of image-guided percutaneous fine needle aspiration biopsy of the mediastinum. Diagn Cytopathol 2007;35(11):705–9.

23. Myojin M, Choi NC, Wright CD, et al. Stage III thymoma: pattern of failure after surgery and postoperative radiotherapy and its implication for future study. Int J Radiat Oncol Biol Phys 2000;46: 927–33.

24. Kim DJ, Yang WI, Choi SS, et al. Prognostic and clinical relevance of the World Health Organization schema for the classification of thymic epithelial tumors: a clinicopathologic study of 108 patients and literature review. Chest 2005;127:755–61.

25. Rea F, Marulli G, Girardi R, et al. Long-term survival and prognostic factors in thymic epithelial tumours. Eur J Cardiothorac Surg 2004;26:412–8.

26. Nakagawa K, Asamura H, Matsuno Y, et al. Thymoma: a clinicopathologic study based on the new World Health Organization classification. J Thorac Cardiovasc Surg 2003;126:1134–40.

27. Regnard JF, Magdeleinat P, Dromer C, et al. Prognostic factors and long-term results after thymoma resection: a series of 307 patients. J Thorac Cardiovasc Surg 1996;112:376–84.

28. Zhu G, He S, Fu X, et al. Radiotherapy and prognostic factors for thymoma: a retrospective study of 175 patients. Int J Radiat Oncol Biol Phys 2004; 60:1113–9.

29. Tomaszek S, Wigle DA, Keshavjee S, et al. Thymomas: review of current clinical practice. Ann Thorac Surg 2009;87:1973–80.

30. Margaritora S, Cesario A, Cusumano G, et al. Thirty-five–year follow-up analysis of clinical and pathologic outcomes of thymoma surgery. Ann Thorac Surg 2010;89:245–52.

31. Phillips LH. The epidemiology of myasthenia gravis. Semin Neurol 2004;24:17–20.

32. Phillips LH II. The epidemiology of myasthenia gravis. Ann N Y Acad Sci 2003;998:407–12.

33. Grob D. Myasthenia gravis-retrospect and prospect. Ann N Y Acad Sci 1981;377:xiii–xxvi.

34. Lindstrom PJ. Autoimmune response to acetylcholine receptor. Science 1973;180:871–2.

35. Keesey JC. A history of treatments for myasthenia gravis. Semin Neurol 2004;24:5–16.

36. Papatestas AE, Genkins G, Kornfeld P, et al. Effects of thymectomy in myasthenia gravis. Ann Surg 1987; 206:79–88.

37. Juel VC, Massey JM. Myasthenia gravis. Orphanet J Rare Dis 2007;2:44.

38. Scherer K, Bedlack RS, Simel DL. Does this patient have myasthenia gravis? JAMA 2005;293: 1906–14.

39. Benatar M. A systematic review of diagnostic studies in myasthenia gravis. Neuromuscul Disord 2006;16:459–67.

40. Vincent A, Newsom-Davis J. Acetylcholine receptor antibody characteristics in myasthenia gravis. III. Patients with low anti-AChR antibody levels. Clin Exp Immunol 1985;60:631–6.

41. Barhon RJ, McIntire D, Herbelin L, et al. Reliability testing of the quantitative myasthenia gravis score. Ann N Y Acad Sci 1998;841:769–72.

42. Myasthenia Gravis Foundation of America recommendations for clinical research standards. In: Kaminski HJ, editor. Myasthenia gravis and related disorders. Totowa (NJ): Humana Press; 2003. p. 373–80.

43. Richman DP, Agius MA. Treatment of autoimmune myasthenia gravis. Neurology 2003;61:1652–61.

44. Onodera H. The role of the thymus in the pathogenesis of myasthenia gravis. Tohoku J Exp Med 2005; 207:87–98.

45. Levinson AI, Song D, Gaulton G. The intrathymic pathogenesis of myasthenia gravis. Clin Dev Immunol 2004;11:215–20.

46. Ragheb S, Lisak RP. The thymus and myasthenia gravis. Chest Surg Clin N Am 2001;11:311–27.

47. Santa T, Engel AG, Lambert EH. Histometric study of neuromuscular junction ultrastructure. I. Myasthenia gravis. Neurology 1972;22:71–82.

48. Santa T, Engel AG, Lambert EG. Histometric study of neuromuscular junction ultrastructure. II. Myasthenic syndrome. Neurology 1972;22:370–6.

49. de Kraker M, Kluin J, Renken N, et al. CT and myasthenia gravis: correlation between mediastinal imaging and histopathological findings. Interact Cardiovasc Thorac Surg 2005;4(3):267–71.

50. Sonett JR, Jaretzki A 3rd. Thymectomy for nonthymomatous myasthenia gravis: a critical analysis. Ann N Y Acad Sci 2008;1132:315–28.

51. Newsom-Davis J, Cutter G, Wolfe GI, et al. Status of the thymectomy trial for nonthymomatous myasthenia gravis patients receiving prednisone. Ann N Y Acad Sci 2008;132:344–7.

52. Krech WG, Storey CF, Umiker W. Thymic cysts: review of literature and report of two cases. J Thorac Cardiovasc Surg 1954;27:477–93.

53. Sirivella S, Gielchinsky I, Parsonnet V. Mediastinal thymic cysts: a report of three cases. J Thorac Cardiovasc Surg 1995;110:1771–2.

54. Wilkins KB, Bulkley GB. Thymectomy in the integrated management of myasthenia gravis. Adv Surg 1999;32:105–33.

55. Blalock A, Mason MF, Morgan HJ, et al. Myasthenia gravis and tumors of the thymic region: report of a case in which the tumor was removed. Ann Surg 1939;110:544–61.

56. Blalock A. Thymectomy in the treatment of myasthenia gravis. Report of twenty cases. J Thorac Surg 1944;13:316–39.

57. Kark AE, Kirschner PA. Total thymectomy by the transcervical approach. Br J Surg 1971;58:321–6.

58. Cooper JD, Al-Jilaihawa AN, Pearson FG, et al. An improved technique to facilitate transcervical thymectomy for myasthenia gravis. Ann Thorac Surg 1988;45(3):242–7.

59. de Perrot M, Bril V, McRae K, et al. Impact of minimally invasive transcervical thymectomy on outcome in patients with myasthenia gravis. Eur J Cardiothorac Surg 2003;24:677–83.

60. Bril V, Kojic J, Ilse WK, et al. Long-term clinical outcome after transcervical thymectomy for myasthenia gravis. Ann Thorac Surg 1998;65(6):1520–2.

61. Shrager JB. Extended transcervical thymectomy: the ultimate minimally invasive approach. Ann Thorac Surg 2010;89(6):S2128–34.

62. Landreneau RJ, Dowling RD, Castillo WM, et al. Thoracoscopic resection of an anterior mediastinal tumor. Ann Thorac Surg 1992;54(1):142–4.

63. Yim AP, Ho JK, Chung SS, et al. One hundred and sixty-three consecutive video thoracoscopic procedures: the Hong Kong experience. Aust N Z J Surg 1994;64(10):671–5.

64. Yim AP, Kay RL, Ho JK. Video-assisted thoracoscopic thymectomy for myasthenia gravis. Chest 1995;108:1440–3.

65. Cheng YJ, Kao EL, Chou SH. Videothoracoscopic resection of stage II thymoma: prospective comparison of the results between thoracoscopy and open methods. Chest 2005;128(4):3010–2.

66. Yoshino I, Hashizume M, Shimada M, et al. Thoracoscopic thymomectomy with the da Vinci computer-enhanced surgical system. Thorac Cardiovasc Surg 2001;122(4):783–5.

67. Jaretzki A III, Aarli JA, Kaminski HJ, et al. Preoperative preparation of patients with myasthenia gravis forestalls postoperative respiratory complications after thymectomy. Ann Thorac Surg 2003; 75:1068.

68. Seggia JC, Abreu P, Takatani M. Plasmapheresis as preparatory method for thymectomy in myasthenia gravis. Arq Neuropsiquiatr 1995;53:411–5.

69. Yeh JH, Chen WH, Huang KM, et al. Prethymectomy plasmapheresis in myasthenia gravis. J Clin Apheresis 2005;20:217–21.

70. Savitt MA, Gao G, Furnary AP, et al. Application of robotic-assisted techniques to the surgical evaluation and treatment of the anterior mediastinum. Ann Thorac Surg 2005;79:450–5.

71. Rea F, Marulli G, Bortolotti L, et al. Experience with the "da Vinci" robotic system for thymectomy in patients with myasthenia gravis: report of 33 cases. Ann Thorac Surg 2006;81:455–9.

72. Wagner AJ, Cortes RA, Strober J, et al. Long-term follow-up after thymectomy for myasthenia gravis: thoracoscopic vs open. J Pediatr Surg 2006;41: 50–4.

73. Iablonskii PK, Pishchik VG, Nuraliev CM. Comparative assessment of the effectiveness of traditional and videothoracoscopic thymectomies in complex treatment of myasthenic thymomas. Vestn Khir Im I I Grek 2005;164:38–42.

74. Hiratsuka M, Iwasaki A, Shirakusa T, et al. Role of video-assisted thoracic surgery for the treatment of myasthenia gravis: extended thymectomy by median sternotomy versus the thoracoscopic approach with sternal lifting. Int Surg 2006;91: 44–51.

75. Toker A, Eroglu O, Ziyade S, et al. Comparison of early postoperative results of thymectomy: partial sternotomy vs. videothoracoscopy. Thorac Cardiovasc Surg 2005;53:110–3.

76. Lin TS, Tzao C, Lee SC, et al. Comparison between video-assisted thoracoscopic thymectomy and transsternal thymectomy for myasthenia gravis (analysis of 82 cases). Int Surg 2005;90:36–41.

77. Augustin F, Schmid T, Sieb M, et al. Video-assisted thoracoscopic surgery versus robotic-assisted thoracoscopic surgery thymectomy. Ann Thorac Surg 2008;85(2):S768–71.

78. Chang PC, Chou SH, Kao EL, et al. Bilateral video-assisted thoracoscopic thymectomy vs. extended transsternal thymectomy in myasthenia gravis: a prospective study. Eur Surg Res 2005;37: 199–203.

79. Bodner J, Wykypiel H, Greiner A, et al. Early experience with robot-assisted surgery for mediastinal masses. Ann Thorac Surg 2004 Jul;78(1): 259–65.

80. Cakar F, Werner P, Augustin F, et al. A comparison of outcomes after robotic open extended thymectomy for myasthenia gravis. Eur J Cardiothorac Surg 2007;31:501–4.

81. Ruckert JC, Ismail M, Swierzy M, et al. Thoracoscopic thymectomy with the da Vinci robotic system for myasthenia gravis. Ann N Y Acad Sci 2008;1132: 329–35.

82. Fleck T, Fleck M, Müller M, et al. Extended videoscopic robotic thymectomy with the da Vinci telemanipulator for the treatment of myasthenia gravis: the Vienna experience. Interact Cardiovasc Thorac Surg 2009;9(5):784–7.

83. Goldstein SD, Yang SC. Assessment of robotic thymectomy using the Myasthenia Gravis Foundation of America Guidelines. Ann Thorac Surg 2010; 89(4):1080–5.

84. Castle SL, Kernstine KH. Robotic-assisted thymectomy. Semin Thorac Cardiovasc Surg 2008;20(4): 326–31.

85. Augustin F, Schmid T, Bodner J. The robotic approach for mediastinal lesions. Int J Med Robot 2006;2(3):262–70.

86. Peliukhovskii SV. [Application of videothoracoscopy in surgical treatment of thymoma and histological characteristics of the tumor]. Klin Khir 2001;54–5 [in Russian].

87. Roviaro G, Varoli F, Nucca O, et al. Videothoraco-scopic approach to primary mediastinal pathology. Chest 2000;117:1179–83.

88. Tarrado X, Ribo JM, Sepulveda JA, et al. Thoraco-scopic thymectomy. Cir Pediatr 2004;17:55–7.

89. Cheng YJ, Wu HH, Chou SH, et al. Video-assisted thoracoscopic management of mediastinal tumors. J Soc Laparoendosc Surg 2001;5:241–4.

90. Cheng YJ, Hsu JS, Kao EL. Characteristics of thy-moma successfully resected by videothoracoscopic surgery. Surg Today 2007;37(3):192–6.

91. Cheng YJ. Videothoracoscopic resection of encap-sulated thymic carcinoma: retrospective compar-ison of the results between thoracoscopy and open methods. Ann Surg Oncol 2008;15(8): 2235–8.

Surgical Management of Stage III Thymic Tumors

Federico Venuta, MD[a],*, Erino A. Rendina, MD[b],
Walter Klepetko, MD[c], Gaetano Rocco, MD[d]

KEYWORDS

- Thymic tumors • Surgical management • Stage III

Epithelial thymic tumors (thymoma and thymic carcinoma) are the most frequent mediastinal tumors in the adult population. This is a heterogeneous group of neoplasm with many unpredictable faces, from an indolent presentation to locally infiltrative and metastasizing lesions. Staging and histology are the most important prognostic factors as is completeness of resection. Many classifications and staging systems have been proposed in the past, both for thymoma and thymic carcinoma, and also an attempt to use the TNM system has been performed without success.[1,2] The only system that has stood the test of time is the one reported by Masaoka and colleagues[3] in 1981 and subsequently modified by Koga and colleagues[4] in 1994. This staging system is based on the evaluation of the local aggressiveness of the tumor (macroscopic and microscopic invasion of the capsule; involvement of the adjacent organs) and the potential lymphatic or hematologic spreading inside or outside the chest (**Table 1**). This classification is easy to assess even at time of surgery and allows an effective prediction of outcome.

Thymic tumors are classified as stage III when they clearly invade the surrounding structures: pericardium, great vessels (superior vena cava [SVC], innominate veins, ascending aorta, and main pulmonary artery), lung parenchyma, phrenic nerves, and chest wall. The support of a pathologist is needed concerning the involvement of the mediastinal pleura: if the tumor is simply grossly adherent to this structure, it is staged as IIB, but if it clearly invades the pleura (confirmed histologically), it is stage III. In-between there is a presentation that is a characterized by tight adhesions between the tumor and the pleura itself. Even simple tight adhesion to the mediastinal pleura has been reported as an ominous prognostic factor; it favors a higher recurrence rate within the pleural space. This is probably related to the need to open and resect the involved pleura even if the tumor is simply adherent. For this reason, Haniuda and colleagues[5] suggested modifying the Masaoka stage II by adding a "p" designator to report on the precise status of the mediastinal pleura. In such revision, stage IIp0 is characterized by no adhesions to the mediastinal surface of the pleura, IIp1 tumors show fibrous adhesions without invasion, and IIp2 manifests true pleural infiltration. The authors found an adverse cutoff point at stage IIp1, regardless of whether or not the lesion was IIA or IIB.

PREOPERATIVE EVALUATION OF STAGE III TUMORS

CT imaging may show some difficulties in identifying invasion of adjacent organs and helping to establish a Masaoka stage III tumor before surgery. Subtle invasion of the adjacent organs, such as the pericardium or the lung, may be

[a] Department of Thoracic Surgery, Policlinico Umberto I, University of Rome Sapienza, Cattedra di Chirurgia Toracica, Viale del Policlinico, 00166 Rome, Italy
[b] Department of Thoracic Surgery, Ospedale Sant'Andrea, University of Rome Sapienza, Rome, Italy
[c] Department of Cardiothoracic Surgery, Vienna Medical University, Vienna, Austria
[d] Pascale Foundation, National Cancer Institute, Naples, Italy
* Corresponding author.
E-mail address: federico.venuta@uniroma1.it

Thorac Surg Clin 21 (2011) 85–91
doi:10.1016/j.thorsurg.2010.08.006
1547-4127/11/$ – see front matter © 2011 Elsevier Inc. All rights reserved.

Table 1 Masaoka–Koga staging system	
Stage I	Macroscopically and microscopically completely encapsulated
Stage IIA	Microscopic transcapsular invasion
Stage IIB	Macroscopic invasion into the surrounding mediastinal fat tissue or grossly adherent to but not through the mediastinal pleura
Stage III	Invasion into the neighboring organs
Stage IVA	Pleural or pericardial dissemination
Stage IVB	Lymphogenous or hematogenous metastases

identified only at the time of mediastinal exploration. In many cases, however, invasion of the local organs can be apparent on pretreatment CT imaging, especially if the vessels are clearly encased and the adventitia loses its margins. Larger tumors (>5 cm) that do not clearly demonstrate frank invasion at CT are likely to show at least serious adhesions with the adjacent organs. An elevated hemidiaphragm with a mediastinal mass abutting either on the cardiac border or toward the right or left pulmonary hilum should indicate invasion of the phrenic nerve.

MRI, although more cumbersome and expensive than CT, may be sometimes helpful preoperatively in evaluating neurovascular structures and vascular invasion.[6] Positron emission tomography has been investigated in the diagnosis and preoperative work-up of these patients. Although the use of semiquantitative maximum standardized uptake value can help differentiate between thymoma and thymic carcinoma, this technique has been inconsistent in distinguishing noninvasive from invasive tumors[7]; notwithstanding that many studies support the value of positron emission tomography imaging, it has not yet become standard practice for evaluating thymic tumors.

SURGICAL CONSIDERATIONS FOR STAGE III THYMIC TUMORS

Complete resection should be the goal and is the gold standard to achieving cure for thymic tumors, including both invasive and metastatic disease. If complete resection could not be anticipated after preoperative work-up, patients should undergo induction chemotherapy to improve outcome.[8–13] Extension of the tumor beyond the thymic gland, however, may not be evident before the operation, and surgeons should be prepared to modify their intraoperative strategy and the extent of the resection accordingly.

Median sternotomy is the standard approach for mediastinal tumors. It provides optimal exposure even in the presence of invasion of the adjacent

structures, such as the lung or great vessels.[14,15] The potential advantages of the sternotomic approach include the speed of opening and closing, the sparing of major thoracic muscles, and reduced postoperative pain.[16] The main disadvantages are related to the limited exposure of the posterolateral compartment of the pleural cavities and of the pulmonary hili, along with the potential risk of sternal infections.

As an alternative, a clamshell incision (bilateral anterior thoracotomy with transverse sternotomy) has been proposed for the excision of large tumors extending in both pleural cavities.[14,17] This approach has been reported as an effective alternative to median sternotomy and in patients with tracheostomy; it allows avoiding communication between the anterosuperior mediastinum and the lower cervical region.[18] The main disadvantage includes a higher postoperative pain and an increased risk of noninfectious sternal complications (overriding and pseudoartrosis).[13,19] For these reasons, the use of this approach is still limited to a few cases.

Recently, an extension of the clamshell incision has been proposed[20]: the inverse T approach. It consists of the association of the standard clamshell incision with a partial upper median sternotomy. This approach allows excellent access to the anterosuperior mediastinum and both pulmonary hili and can be easily extended to the cervical region. Despite the extension of the incision, good results in terms of preservation of the chest wall stability and sternocostal arch functionality are reported,[20,21] with fast recovery and early respiratory rehabilitation.

An alternative approach is the thoracosternotomy or hemiclamshell incision that allows greater exposure of one pleural space. This exposure starts with an anterior thoracotomy on the side with the greatest bulk of tumor, entering the chest through the fourth intercostal space. Once feasibility of the resection is determined, the approach is completed with partial median sternotomy from the opened intercostals space upward. The hemithorax is lifted with a retractor of the type used to expose and harvest the internal mammary artery for coronary artery bypass. This incision provides significantly greater exposure than standard median sternotomy, allowing excellent visualization of the brachiocephalic vessels and phrenic nerve, especially with larger tumors; also, upper lobectomy may be accomplished easily through this incision, if required. Closure of this incision proceeds in the same fashion as that for median sternotomy with the additional placement of a few pericostal sutures at the level of the opened intercostals space.[22]

Stage III thymic tumors often provide a major challenge, particularly in patients requiring preoperative induction treatment. If complete resection is accomplished, however, survival rates can be comparable with those of patients with stage I and II disease.[23] The left brachiocephalic vein, SVC, right atrium, pericardium, lung, and diaphragm can be safely resected with or without reconstruction. Also, resection of one phrenic nerve or reconstruction of the ascending aorta and main pulmonary artery may be indicated to achieve complete resection; alternatively, invasion through the pericardium into the myocardium usually precludes resection.

Removal of the anterior pericardium is not routine, but even tight adhesions between a tumor and the pericardial sac may make it difficult to exclude direct invasion; this can also happen in tumors apparently capsulated. Excision of any tightly adherent part of the sac should be accomplished. Reconstruction of the resulting defect is optional; if it is considered, bovine pericardium or any other prosthetic material may be used; also, materials that help prevent the creation of adhesions with the myocardium could be of help[24,25] when resection of a mediastinal recurrence is required in the future or in heart surgery.

Direct invasion into the lung should be resected as allowed by respiratory function. Stapled wedge excision is appropriate in most cases because the tumor usually tends to involve only the anterior segment of the right upper lobe or the lingula; however, segmental resection or anatomic lobectomy may be necessary in cases of deeper invasion. Pneumonectomy or extrapleural pneumonectomy is rarely required but can be performed if the tumor involves the pulmonary hilum or the pleura. These procedures are justified in young and otherwise healthy patients and should be preceded by induction therapy.

The diaphragm is rarely involved by huge thymic tumors; it is most often the site of secondary implants. In both cases, induction chemotherapy should be administered before attempting full-thickness excision and subsequent reconstruction.

The definition of phrenic nerve invasion/injury should be based on clear criteria: (1) description of a phrenic nerve resection en bloc with the tumor within the operatory report, (2) description of a phrenic nerve segment detected during pathologic examination of the surgical specimen, and (3) postoperative chest x-ray finding of an elevated hemidiaphragm in patients without this evidence preoperatively.[26] In patients with reasonably preserved lung function, one phrenic nerve may be sacrificed with relative impunity; however, the resection or damage of both nerves should be avoided because it leaves patients with significant respiratory compromise. If a phrenic nerve is to be sacrificed, consideration should be given to prophylactic diaphragm plication at the time of thymectomy.[22] If the tumor infiltrates both phrenic nerves, as much tumor as possible should be removed while leaving the nerves intact. Care must be taken to avoid compromising the tenuous blood supply to the nerves because it could result in diaphragmatic paralysis.[22] These maneuvers should be more cautious in patients with limited pulmonary reserve and in those affected by myasthenia gravis. In cases where complete resection cannot be achieved because it is prevented by other concurrent problems, debulking (with all the prognostic limitations of this approach) should be performed with preservation of both phrenic nerves.

Vascular reconstructions pose more serious technical problems. Both the SVC and the brachiocephalic veins can be resected and reconstructed but only if that helps achieve complete resection. If the SVC is infiltrated for less than 30% of the circumference, partial resection of the wall of the vessel is usually feasible and repair can be accomplished either by direct suture or patch interposition; autologous material (pericardial or venous) is usually used. If a larger circumferential involvement is present, complete resection of the vessel with prosthetic reconstruction is required. These operations represent a major technical challenge for the potential detrimental effect of clamping a patent vessel[27] and the risk of complications. Partial SVC clamping of a chronically obstructed vessel is usually well tolerated. Alternatively, if complete clamping of a patent SVC is required, a marked hemodynamic imbalance may occur, with consequent increase of the mean venous pressure in the cephalic district and a reduced arteriovenous gradient within the brain. This may result in cerebral edema, hemorrhage, and damage and potentially lethal reduction of cardiac output. The hemodynamic derangement may be limited by a dedicated pharmacologic support and intra- or extraluminal shunt placement.

Full circumferential reconstruction of the SVC can be performed by prosthetic replacement if a disease-free confluence of both the innominate veins is available. To avoid kinking of the prosthesis, the length of the conduit should be adapted so that the distal anastomosis is under moderate tension. In cases of invasion of the SVC at the confluence of the two innominate veins, the reconstruction is usually performed, anastomosing one of the two veins with the inferior SVC stump, closing the contralateral innominate vein; the choice is made on the base of local invasion and anatomic consideration. Usually, the revascularization of both innominate veins implanted independently on the right atrium is not performed because the blood flow through the grafts could be too low and favor the risk of thrombosis. Successful complete resection of the SVC and both innominate veins with subsequent reconstruction with a Y-shaped prosthesis have been reported in the literature[15]; this option should be considered when cervical anastomosis between the two venous systems is not available (previous thyroid cancer surgery and radiotherapy).

These reconstructions are usually realized with synthetic materials (rigid polytetrafluoroethylene grafts) or bovine pericardium. The latter displays some advantageous characteristics, such as the presence of even and stiff edges and a limited tendency to retract.[28] Among the synthetic materials, polytetrafluoroethylene is the most frequently used because it shows the highest long term patency rate and, shortly after implantation, it becomes re-epithelialized with autologous cells.

Autologous venous grafts show a limited diameter that may be sufficient only to reconstruct the left brachiocephalic vein but not the entire SVC. A saphenous vein graft of adequate diameter, however, has been created by suturing the vessel in a spiral fashion around an adequate support (usually a chest drainage or a syringe).[29]

Patch reconstruction is usually accomplished with biologic materials. Autologous pericardium has been extensively used because it shows several advantages: it has adequate thickness and resistance to pressure and tension; it is cost-free; harvesting does not require a separate surgical procedure or approach; it is able to offer a larger amount of viable tissue when compared with venous patches; and it is also available with a lateral thoracotomy approach. The autologous pericardium, however, shows some technical limitation because it tends to shrink and curl, making sizing more difficult. For this reason, it has been suggested an original method of fixation of the patch with glutaraldehyde[30]; this method allows obtaining stiff edges and no tendency to shrink and curl, making tailoring much easier.

Difficult situations with intracaval–intra-atrial involvement of the SVC require an aggressive approach with the institution of cardiopulmonary bypass.[31–34] Also, en bloc resection of the ascending aorta and pulmonary vessels has been reported in a few cases.[35–37] Although technically feasible, it should be considered only to achieve complete resection and it is considered a negative prognostic factor.[38] These procedures are performed under cardiopulmonary bypass and, in some of them, circulatory arrest and retrograde brain perfusion are required, in particular when the aortic arch is to be reconstructed.[35]

RESULTS

The impact on survival of surgical resection of stage III thymic tumors is difficult to be assessed because in most of the series the operation is associated either to induction chemotherapy[8–12,39] or postoperative adjuvant treatment.[5,23,40–44] The 5-year survival rates are encouraging, however, although local and distant recurrence still exists. Survival at 5 years at this stage ranges from 46%[45] to 88%[23]; at 10 years it ranges from 26%[46] to 84%.[47] This wide variability is mainly related to the inclusion of patients undergoing partial resection and the variable administration of induction and adjuvant treatment. Surgery alone is rarely the only treatment modality. In all the reported studies, there is an uniform agreement about considering completeness of resection as a key factor for success, especially at this stage.[23,38,48–55] Patients with R0 stage III thymoma after surgery show survival rates similar to those with stage I tumors. This observation implies that the ability to achieve complete resection may be the most important prognostic factor; this was observed at multivariate analysis in a group of 307 patients; in that study, complete resection was the only significant prognostic factor (stage was not significant if completeness of resection was included in the model).[48] This finding should encourage an aggressive surgical approach and the need to administer induction therapy when complete resection cannot be anticipated at preoperative work-up; this treatment modality is certainly able to increase the complete resection rate.[8–12,39] It has been reported that completeness of resection loses its statistical significance in a group of patients receiving the multimodality approach (including induction and adjuvant treatment).[10] This finding has not been observed, however, by other groups[9,12]; this might be related to the small number of patients included in each study. This observation has been justified with the hypothesis that with the combined modality treatment, complete resection becomes less crucial because the goal of complete tumoral clearance is achieved by the whole treatment.[10] Also, postoperative radiotherapy on a small residual mass may be more effective after induction and in concurrence with adjuvant chemotherapy, allowing complete clearance of the bed of the tumor. This finding might encourage revising the staging system, giving more weight to the GETT classification, although it could only play a role postoperatively.

A systematic review has been performed to investigate the role of surgery in the management of thymic tumors.[56] The study was based on a literature search on articles published in English between 1981 and 2007. The final analysis included a single, prospective, randomized controlled trial and 23 retrospective series with between 40 and 1093 patients; patients included in these studies were subjected to various combinations of surgery, radiotherapy, and chemotherapy. The use of surgery as the sole therapeutic maneuver depends on the stage considered. Evidence-based treatment recommendations for stage III thymoma are reported as follows:

- The surgeon should strive to completely resect stage III thymomas becuase complete resection increases survival (C1: methods weak; effect clear).
- Subtotal resection followed by adjuvant treatment may be undertaken in the belief that it will prolong survival (C2: methods weak; effect equivocal).
- Stage III thymomas should be resected by median sternotomy to achieve maximal exposure and maximally enable intraoperative macroscopic staging (C2: methods weak; effect clear).

In most of the studies, however, the decision to add adjuvant treatment was not driven by protocols; thus, significant selection bias was likely present.

In conclusion, surgical resection still plays a critical role in the treatment of stage III thymic tumors and should be the first choice when complete resection can be anticipated at preoperative work-up. In cases of bulky invasive tumors, induction chemotherapy can contribute to reduce the volume of the mass, downstage the lesion, and eventually achieve complete resection. Adjuvant treatment is recommended in cases of incomplete resection or simple debulking; its role after complete resection should be validated with prospective randomized studies.

REFERENCES

1. Yamakawa Y, Masaoka A, Hoshimoto T, et al. A tentative tumor—node metastasis classification of thymoma. Cancer 1991;68:1984—7.
2. International Union Against Cancer. TNM supplement. A commentary on uniform use. 3rd edition. New York: Wiley—Liss; 2003.
3. Masaoka A, Monden Y, Nakahara K, et al. Follow up study of thymomas with special reference to their clinical stages. Cancer 1981;48:2485—92.
4. Koga K, Matsuno Y, Noguchi M, et al. A review of 78 thymomas: modification of staging system and reappraisal of conventional division into invasive and non invasive thymoma. Pathol Int 1994;44:359—67.
5. Haniuda M, Morimoto M, Nishimura H, et al. Adjuvant radiotherapy after complete resection of thymoma. Ann Thorac Surg 1992;54:311—5.
6. Rosado-de-Christenson ML, Strollo DC, Marom EM. Imaging of thymic epithelial neoplasms. Hematol Oncol Clin North Am 2008;22:409—31.
7. Puri V, Meyers BF. Utility of positron emission tomography in the mediastinum: moving beyond lung and esophageal cancer staging. Thorac Surg Clin 2009;19:7—15.
8. Venuta F, Rendina EA, Pescarmona E, et al. Multimodality treatment of thymorna: a prospective study. Ann Thorac Surg 1997;64:1585—92.
9. Venuta F, Rendina EA, Longo F, et al. Long term out come after multimodality treatment for stage III thymic tumors. Ann Thorac Surg 2003;76:1866—72.
10. Lucchi M, Ambrogi MC, Duranti L, et al. Advanced stage thymomas and thymic carcinomas: results of multimodality treatment. Ann Thorac Surg 2005;79:1840—4.
11. Macchiarini P, Chella A, Ducci F, et al. Neoadjuvant chemotherapy, surgery and postoperative radiation therapy for invasive thymoma. Cancer 1991;68:706—13.
12. Kim ES, Putnam JB, Komaki R, et al. Phase II study of a multidisciplinary approach with induction chemotherapy followed by surgical resection, radiation therapy and consolidation chemotherapy for unresectable malignant thymomas: final report. Lung Cancer 2004;44:369—79.
13. Wright C. Transverse sternothoracotomy. Chest Surg Clin N Am 1996;6:149—56.
14. Bacha EA, Chapelier AR, Macchiarini P, et al. Surgery for invasive primary mediastinal tumors. Ann Thorac Surg 1998;66:234—8.
15. Chen KN, Xu SF, Gu ZD, et al. Surgical treatment of complex malignant anterior mediastinal tumors invading the superior vena cava. World J Surg 2006;30:162—70.
16. Cooper JD, Nelems JM, Pearson FG. Extended indications for median sternotomy in patients requiring

pulmonary resection. Ann Thorac Surg 1978;26:
413–20.

17. Bains MS, Ginsberg RJ, Jones WG 3rd, et al. The clamshell incision: an improved approach to bilateral pulmonary and mediastinal tumors. Ann Thorac Surg 1994;58:30–3.

18. Marshall WG Jr, Meng RL, Ehrenhaft JL. Coronary artery bypass grafting in patients with a tracheostoma: use of a bilateral thoracotomy incision. Ann Thorac Surg 1988;46:465–6.

19. Brown RP, Esmore DS, Lawson C. Improved sternal fixation in the transsternal bilateral thoracotomy incision. J Thorac Cardiovasc Surg 1996;112:137–41.

20. Marta GM, Aigner C, Klepetko W. Inverse T incision provides improved accessibility to the upper mediastinum. J Thorac Cardiovasc Surg 2005; 129:221–3.

21. Aigner C, Hoda MAR, Klepetko W. Combined cervicothoracic approaches for complex mediastinal masses. Thorac Surg Clin 2009;19:107–12.

22. Kaiser LR. Surgical treatment of thymic epithelial neoplasms. Hematol Oncol Clin North Am 2008;22: 175–88.

23. Nakahara K, Ohno K, Hashimoto J, et al. Thymoma: results with complete resection and adjuvant postoperative irradiation in 141 consecutive patients. J Thorac Cardiovasc Surg 1988;95:1041–7.

24. Pace Napoleone C, Oppido G, Angeli E, et al. Resternotomy in pediatric cardiac surgery: CoSeal initial experience. Interact Cardiovasc Thorac Surg 2007; 6:21–3.

25. Pace Napoleone C, Valori A, Crupi G, et al. An observational study of CoSeal for the prevention of adhesions in pediatric cardiac surgery. Interact Cardiovasc Thorac Surg 2009;9:979–82.

26. Salati M, Cardillo G, Carbone L, et al. Iatrogenic phrenic nerve injury during thymectomy: the extent of the problem. J Thorac Cardiovasc Surg 2010; 139:77–8.

27. Gonzalez-Fajado JA, Garcia-Juste M, Florez S, et al. Hemodynamic cerebral repercussions arising from surgical interruption of the superior vena cava. Experimental model. J Thorac Cardiovasc Surg 1994;107:1044–9.

28. D'Andrilli A, Ciccone AM, Ibrahim M, et al. A new technique for prosthetic reconstruction of the superior vena cava. J Thorac Cardiovasc Surg 2006; 132:192–4.

29. Doty DB. By pass of superior vena cava: six years experience with spiral vein graft for obstruction of superior vena cava due to benign and malignant disease. J Thorac Cardiovasc Surg 1982;83: 326–9.

30. D'Andrilli A, Ibrahim M, Vanuta F, et al. Glutaraldehide preserved autologous pericardium for patch roconotruotion of the pulmonary artery and superior vena cava. Ann Thorac Surg 2005;80:357–8.

31. Minato N, Rikitake K, Ohnishi H, et al. Invasive thymoma with intracaval growth extending and directly invading the right atrium. J Cardiovasc Surg 1999; 40:915–7.

32. De Giacomo T, Mazzesi G, Venuta F, et al. Extended operation for recurrent thymic carcinoma presenting with intracaval growth and intracardiac extension. J Thorac Cardiovasc Surg 2007;134:1364–5.

33. Kostantinov IE, Saxena P, Koniszko M, et al. Superior vena cava obstruction by tumor thrombus in invasive thymoma: diagnosis and surgical management. Heart Lung Circ 2007;16:462–4.

34. Amirghogran AA, Ememinia A, Rayatpisheh S, et al. Intracardiac invasive thymoma presenting as superior vena cava syndrome. Ann Thorac Surg 2009; 87:1616–8.

35. Fujino S, Teruke N, Watorida S, et al. Reconstruction of the aortic arch in invasive thymoma under retrograde cerebral perfusion. Ann Thorac Surg 1998; 66:263–4.

36. Tseng YL, Wang ST, Wu MH, et al. Thymic carcinoma: involvement of great vessels indicates poor prognosis. Ann Thorac Surg 2003;76:1041–5.

37. Park BJ, Bacchetta M, Mains MS, et al. Surgical management of thoracic malignancies invading the heart or great vessels. Ann Thorac Surg 2004;78: 1024–30.

38. Okumura M, Miyoshi S, Takeuchi Y, et al. Results of surgical treatment of thymomas with special reference to the involved organs. J Thorac Cardiovasc Surg 1999;117:605–11.

39. Rea F, Sartori F, Loy M, et al. Chemotherapy and operation for invasive thymoma. J Thorac Cardiovasc Surg 1993;106:543–9.

40. Urghesi A, Monetti U, Rossi G, et al. Role of radiation therapy in locally advanced thymoma. Radiother Oncol 1990;19:273–80.

41. Jackson MA, Mall DL. Postoperative radiotherapy in invasive thymoma. Radiother Oncol 1991;21: 77–82.

42. Latz D, Schraube P, Oppiz U, et al. Invasive thymoma: treatment with postoperative radiation therapy. Radiology 1997;204:859–64.

43. Gripp S, Hilgers K, Wurm R, et al. Thymoma: prognostic factors and treatment outcomes. Cancer 1988;83:1495–503.

44. Ogawa K, Uno T, Toita T, et al. Postoperative radiotherapy for patients with completely resected thymoma. Cancer 2002;94:1405–13.

45. Elert O, Buchwald J, Wolf K. Epithelial thymic tumors—therapy and prognosis. Thorac Cardiovasc Surg 1988;36:109–13.

46. Blumberg D, Burt ME, Bains MS, et al. Thymic carcinoma: current staging does not predict prognosis. J Thorac Cardiovasc Surg 1998;115:303–9.

47. Strobel P, Bauer A, Puppe B, et al. Tumor recurrence and survival in patients treated for thymomas and

thymic squamous cell carcinomas: a retrospective analysis. J Clin Oncol 2004;22:1501–9.

48. Regnard JF, Magdeleinat P, Dromer C, et al. Prognostic factors and long term results after thymoma resection. A series of 307 patients. J Thorac Cardiovasc Surg 1996;112:376–84.

49. Lewis JE, Wick MR, Scheithaner BW, et al. Thymoma: a clinicopathologic review. Cancer 1987;60: 2727–43.

50. Maggi G, Casadio C, Cavallo A, et al. Thymoma: results of 241 operated cases. Ann Thorac Surg 1991;51:152–6.

51. Okumura M, Ohta M, Tateyama H, et al. The World Health Organization histologic classification system reflects the oncologic behaviour of thymoma: a clinical study of 273 patients. Cancer 2002;94:624–32.

52. Wilkins KB, Sheikh E, Green R, et al. Clinical and pathologic predictors of survival in patients with thymoma. Ann Surg 1999;230:562–74.

53. Blumberg D, Port JL, Wechsler B, et al. Thymoma: a multivariate analysis of factors predicting survival. Ann Thorac Surg 1995;60:908–14.

54. Rea F, Marulli G, Girardi R, et al. Long term serival and prognostic factors in thymic epithelial tumors. Eur J Cardiothorac Surg 2004;26:412–8.

55. Myojin M, Choi NC, Wright CD, et al. Stage III thymoma: pattern of failure after surgery and postoperative radiotherapy and its implication for future study. Int J Radiat Oncol Biol Phys 2000;46:927–33.

56. Davenport E, Malthaner RA. The role of surgery in the management of thymoma: a systematic review. Ann Thorac Surg 2008;86:673–84.

Stage IVA Thymoma: Patterns of Spread and Surgical Management

Cameron D. Wright, MD

KEYWORDS

- Thymoma • Pleural disease • Pleurectomy
- Pleuropneumonectomy

Almost all series reporting on the results of resection in thymic tumors indicate that the performance of a complete resection is probably the most important prognostic factor.[1] This issue is not a factor in Masaoka stage I and II tumors, which are almost always easily completely resected and have an excellent prognosis. Masaoka stage III tumors, which invade the pericardium, lung, or great vessels, have higher incomplete resection rates, significantly higher recurrence rates, and thus a worse prognosis.[1–3] Masaoka stage IVA tumors represent intrapleural spread of thymoma tumor cells to a favored biologic host site—the pleura. The reason for this unique behavior is unknown. Pleural metastases can be present at the original presentation of the thymoma or be detected as recurrent disease. Intrapleural relapse is the most common site of relapse of resected thymomas.[2–5] The most common areas of relapse tend to be the paravertebral gutter and the diaphragm (**Figs. 1 and 2**). Treatment options include local pleural resection, total pleurectomy, pleuropneumonectomy, chemotherapy, intrapleural chemotherapy or photodynamic therapy, and radiation. The management of pleural recurrences has been recently reviewed by Lucchi and colleagues.[6]

RECURRENCE PATTERNS AFTER THYMOMA RESECTION

Recurrences can be local (mediastinal), pleural, or distant after thymoma resection. Lung, followed by liver, and then bone are the most common distant metastatic sites—all of which are rare.[2–5] Local recurrences are surprisingly uncommon. The most common site of recurrence in essentially all large series is the pleural space, ranging from 46% to 80% of all recurrences (**Table 1**).[2–5] Several reports have noted the time to relapse, ranging from 29 to 42 and to 60 months.[3,5,6] One report stratified time to recurrence according to stage: stage I or II—8.5 years, stage III—5 years, and stage IVA—3.5 years.[3] One report stratified time to recurrence according to histology: thymoma (29 months) and thymic carcinoma (9 months).[5] This information has guided the author's follow-up of these patients with pleural spread. Thymic carcinoma patients have a surveillance chest CT every 6 months whereas thymoma patients have a yearly CT for follow-up.

INDUCTION THERAPY FOR PLEURAL DISEASE

Pleural dissemination represents advanced disease and is not amenable to a true en bloc resection. Accordingly, most investigators have promoted using chemotherapy, usually as an induction agent but also in an adjuvant fashion to attempt to enhance progression-free survival in association with pleural resection. There are no prospective studies to guide management leading to institutional preferences for treatment plans. The author's preference is to use the pleural disease as measurable disease to test chemotherapy responsiveness to find an effective regimen if possible. Resection is then performed after 2 to 4 cycles according to the response. The

Division of Thoracic Surgery, Department of Surgery, Massachusetts General Hospital, Harvard Medical School, Boston, MA 02114, USA
E-mail address: cdwright@partners.org

Thorac Surg Clin 21 (2011) 93–97
doi:10.1016/j.thorsurg.2010.08.007

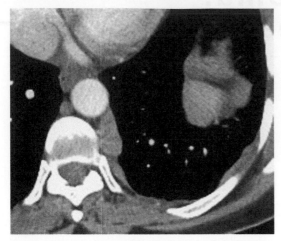

Fig. 1. CT scan of an isolated parietal pleural metastases from a recurrent B2 thymoma after resection in the left paravertebral gutter. A local pleurectomy was done after chemotherapy.

two most common regimens used are cisplatin, doxorubicin, and cyclophosphamide (PAC) and cisplatin, doxorubicin, vincristine, and cyclophosphamide (ADOC).[7,8] Although the author's group has favored induction chemoradiotherapy for locally advanced thymic tumors, they rarely use that approach with extensive pleural disease due to lung toxicity concerns.[9] Recurrent thymoma is usually an indolent disease, and sometimes careful observation is wise before deciding on any aggressive treatment depending on patient characteristics.

PLEURECTOMY FOR PLEURAL DISEASE

Local or total pleurectomy has been done for many years for pleural disease. Recently, several series have been reported, focusing on the results of pleurectomy (**Table 2**).[10–12] Most pleural metastases are limited in number, distribution, and depth

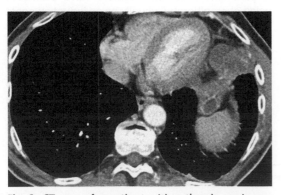

Fig. 2. CT scan of a patient with a thymic carcinoma and multiple pleural metastases localized to the anterior diaphragmatic sulcus.

of invasion, leading to relatively easy local pleurectomy by a posterolateral thoracotomy. Most surgeons favor resecting the macroscopic disease and do not do a total pleurectomy, as is done in mesothelioma. Which strategy is optimal is unknown. Repeat pleurectomy has been reported after the initial pleural resection with apparent benefit.[10,12]

PLEUROPNEUMONECTOMY FOR EXTENSIVE IVA DISEASE

Extensive, often confluent, pleural disease is usually also associated with widespread lung invasion and requires pleuropneumonectomy for near complete resection. Although at first glance this seems like heroic surgery, the biology of this tumor with long survival even with a recurrence favors an aggressive approach. Many case reports have demonstrated the feasibility of this concept. More recently, several small series have been reported that demonstrate reasonable results (**Table 3**).[11–13] Although a true en bloc complete resection cannot be performed, the amount of disease that is left is typically not visible and truly microscopic. Most cases require resection of the ipsilateral pericardium and diaphragm as well, similar to that of mesothelioma resection. Typically, induction chemotherapy is given before resection to maximize any possible downstaging. Radiation should rarely be given as an induction agent because the lung and pleura are removed and the involved field is large, leading to increased toxicity. Radiation is typically given as an adjuvant for any areas the surgeon had a concern for intraoperatively. Similar to mesothelioma treatment, it is easier and safer to give radiation to the hemithorax once the lung is removed.

TECHNIQUE OF PLEUROPNEUMONECTOMY FOR EXTENSIVE STAGE IVA DISEASE

The preoperative cardiopulmonary evaluation should be thorough in patients who require pleuropneumonectomy because a pneumonectomy is a significant physiologic insult. Complete pulmonary function tests, a quantitative ventilation perfusion scan if lung function is abnormal, an echocardiogram, and a stress test if there is any suspicion of coronary disease are the standard tests. A positron emission tomography/CT is helpful to eliminate the possibility of extrathoracic disease before this major resection. Most surgeons use a posterolateral thoracotomy for the operative approach. Others have described a median sternotomy approach or a clamshell/hemiclamshell approach.[13] In large part, this

Table 1
Pleural relapse after thymoma resection

Author, Year	No. of Patients	Pleural	Local	Distant
Regnard, 1996	307	14 (56%)	10	1
Wright, 2005	179	16 (80%)	2	2
Utsumi, 2008	84 Stage III	12 (46%)	6	8
Huang, 2009	97	8 (53%)	5	2

revolves around the extent of the mediastinal component of the tumor, with larger tumors benefiting from anterior access rather than lateral access.

Typical patients are resected via a large posterolateral thoracotomy with division of both the latisimus and the serratus anterior muscles.[14] Usually the sixth rib is resected to enhance access. Often a lower thoracotomy is done under the divided latisimus to enhance access to the diaphragm if needed. The subpleural plane is entered bluntly with the surgeon's fingers and a complete resection of the parietal pleura is done off the anterior, lateral, and posterior chest walls. The mediastinal pleura is dissected next with care to avoid injury to important mediastinal structures, such as the vagus, aorta and arch vessels, esophagus, and azygos vein. The pericardium is entered at its periphery and resected as well. The artery and two veins to the lung are stapled and divided followed by the bronchus. The diaphragm is usually resected. If so, and if there is minimal diaphragm involvement, it is useful to maintain the peritoneum relatively intact. The diaphragm is reconstructed with PTFE with anchoring to the chest wall with nonabsorbable sutures. The pericardium is reconstructed with PTFE with fenestrations or with absorbable mesh.

RESULTS OF PLEUROPNEUMONECTOMY FOR EXTENSIVE STAGE IVA DISEASE

The results of pleuropneumonectomy are good despite the aggressive nature of the operation

(**Fig. 3**).[11–13] The perioperative morbidity and mortality that have been reported are low and probably reflect in part careful patient selection and also an absence of smoking on the patient population (see **Table 3**). The reported 5-year survival in the three larger series, approximately 75%, is remarkable (see **Table 3**).[11–13] Caution is in order, however, because many recurrences occur after 5 years and there is usually a long time between recurrence and death. Nonetheless, these results seem to justify this aggressive approach to this rare subset of thymic tumor patients.

NOVEL TREATMENTS FOR PLEURAL RECURRENCES

There has always been concern for a close microscopic margin after pleurectomy for pleural thymoma, regardless of whether or not it was partial, total, or done with an extrapleural pneumonectomy. A topical treatment for this presumably limited microscopic disease seems rational. De Bree and colleagues[15] reported on the use of intraoperative hyperthermic chemotherapy after cytoreductive surgery for either mesothelioma or thymoma. There has been significant worldwide interest in this concept for mesothelioma, ovarian cancer, and, more recently, stage IVA thymoma. Studies have shown less systemic absorption and higher local concentrations of chemotherapeutic agents.[16] Long-term results are awaited. Likewise, photodynamic therapy has been investigated for mesothelioma and found possible.[17] Initial studies are under

Table 2
Results of pleurectomy in stage IVA disease

Author, Year	No. of Patients	Induction	Mortality	Survival
Huang, 2007	14	PAC	0	5 NED, 7 AWD, 2 DOD
Ishkawa, 2009	7	6/7, CAMP	0	2 NED, 4 AWD, 2 TRD
Lucchi, 2009	20	None, 7 adjuvant	0	43% 5 year

Abbreviations: AWD, alive with disease; CAMP, cisplatin, doxorubicin, and methylprednisolone; DOD, dead of disease; NED, no evidence of disease; TRD, treatment-related death.

Table 3
Results of pleuropneumonectomy for stage IVA disease

Author, Year	No. of Patients, Thymoma with Cancer	Induction Therapy	Mortality	Adjuvant Therapy	Survival
Wright, 2006	5, All B3	2/5	0	5/5	75% 5 year
Huang, 2007	4, All thymomas	4/4	0	4/4	78% 5 year
Ishikawa, 2009	4, All thymomas	4/4	0	3/4	75% 5 year

way investigating the role of photodynamic therapy in stage IVA thymoma.

PROGNOSTIC FACTORS IN STAGE IVA THYMOMA

There is limited information on prognostic factors after treatment of stage IVA thymoma because there are few patients in any given report. Two reports have reported on univariate prognostic factors with pleural disease. Lucchi and colleagues[10] found single pleural implants (vs multiple) were more favorable. In addition, diaphragmatic involvement was associated with a worse prognosis. Ishikawa and colleagues[12] reported that patients who had a pleuropneumonectomy as opposed to local pleural resection had a more favorable prognosis.

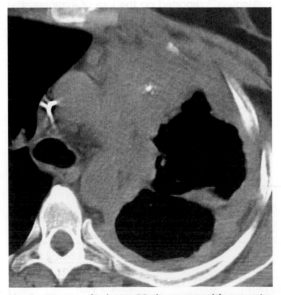

Fig. 3. CT scan of a large B3 thymoma with extensive lung and pleural involvement, which required pleuropneumonectomy for resection.

REFERENCES

1. Venuta F, Anile M, Disco D, et al. Thymoma and thymic carcinoma. Eur J Cardiothorac Surg 2010; 37:13–25.
2. Wright CD, Wain JC, Wong DR, et al. Predictors of recurrence in thymic tumors: importance of invasion, WHO histology and size. J Thorac Cardiovasc Surg 2005;130:1413–21.
3. Regnard JF, Magdeleinant P, Dromer C, et al. Prognostic factors and long-term results after thymoma resection; a series of 307 patients. J Thorac Cardiovasc Surg 1996;112:376–84.
4. Utsumi T, Shiono S, Matsumura A, et al. Stage III thymoma: relationship of local invasion to recurrence. J Thorac Cardiovasc Surg 2008;136:1481–5.
5. Huang J, Rizik NP, Travis WD, et al. Comparison of patterns of relapse in thymic carcinoma and thymoma. J Thorac Cardiovasc Surg 2009;138:26–31.
6. Lucchi M, Basolo F, Mussi A. Surgical management of pleural recurrence from thymoma. Eur J Cardiothorac Surg 2008;33:707–11.
7. Casey EM, Kiel PJ, Loehrer PJ. Clinical management of thymma patients. Hematol Oncol Clin North Am 2008;22:409–31.
8. Venuta F, Rendina EA, Longo F, et al. Long-term outcome after multimodality treatment for treatment of stage III thymic tumors. Ann Thorac Surg 2003; 76:1866–72.
9. Wright CD, Choi NC, Wain JC, et al. Induction chemoradiotherapy followed by resection for locally advanced Masaoka stage III and IVA thymic tumors. Ann Thorac Surg 2008;85:385–9.
10. Lucchi M, Davini F, Ricciardi R, et al. Management of pleural recurrence after curative resection of thymoma. J Thorac Cardiovasc Surg 2009;137:1185–9.
11. Huang J, Rizk NP, Travis WD, et al. Feasability of multimodality therapy including extended resections in stage IVA thymoma. J Thorac Cardiovasc Surg 2007;134:1477–84.
12. Ishikawa Y, Matsuguma H, Nakahara R, et al. Multimodality therapy for patients with invasive thymoma disseminated into the pleural cavity; the potential

role of extrapleural pneumonectomy. Ann Thorac Surg 2009;88:952–7.

13. Wright CD. Pleuropneumonectomy for the treatment of Masaoka Stage IVA thymoma. Ann Thorac Surg 2006;82:1234–9.

14. Chang MY, Sugarbaker DJ. Extrapleural pneumonectomy for diffuse malignant mesothelioma: techniques and complications. Thorac Surg Clin 2004; 14:523–30.

15. De Bree E, van Ruth S, Baas P, et al. Cytoreductive surgery and intraoperative hyperthermic chemotherapy in patients with malignant mesothelioma or pleural metastases of thymoma. Chest 2002;121:480–7.

16. De Bree E, van Ruth S, Schotborgh CE, et al. Limited cardiotoxicity after extensive thoracic surgery and intraoperative hyperthermic chemotherapy with doxorubicin and cisplatin. Ann Surg Oncol 2007; 14:319–26.

17. Rodriguez E, Baas P, Friedberg JS. Innovative therapies: Photodynamic therapy. Thorac Surg Clin 2004;14:557–66.

The Role of Radiotherapy in the Management of Thymic Tumors

Nicolas Girard, MD[a,b,c], Françoise Mornex, MD, PhD[a,c],*

KEYWORDS

- Thymoma • Thymic carcinoma • Radiotherapy
- Chemotherapy • Surgery

Thymic tumors are rare intrathoracic cancers that represent 0.2% to 1.5% of all malignancies and that may be aggressive and difficult to treat.[1,2] Histopathologically, these tumors are classified as thymomas (types A, AB, B1, B2, and B3) or thymic carcinomas.[3] Clinically, invasion or tumor stage, as per the standard Masaoka classification, is a major prognostic factor of overall survival.[4] Surgery is the cornerstone of management of thymomas, initially being useful for precise diagnosis and staging, and in most cases ensuring the first step of the therapeutics simultaneously.[2,5] The most significant prognostic factor is then whether the tumor can be completely resected at surgery.[5,6]

In general, thymomas are tumors with a tendency toward local recurrence rather than metastasis. Thus, thymomas historically have been treated surgically, possibly followed by radiotherapy.[2,5] By contrast, thymic carcinomas have a high risk of relapse and death despite surgery, chemotherapy, and radiotherapy.[2,7]

Because of their rarity, knowledge about thymic tumors has been based on small retrospective series for a long time. More recently, evidence-based guidelines have been designed by several collaborative groups internationally.[2,8–11] Meta-analyses have been performed to support these recommendations, especially regarding the role of radiotherapy.[12] As discussed in this article, the role of radiotherapy, given as adjuvant, neoadjuvant, or exclusive treatment, is one of the most debated issues in the management of thymic tumors.

RADIOTHERAPY FOR THYMIC TUMORS: TECHNIQUES
Conformal Radiotherapy

Most studies reporting about the management of thymic tumors are retrospective. Data regarding radiotherapy are highly heterogeneous,[12] given the long-term recruitment periods and considering the significant improvements in radiation delivery techniques that were observed over the past 20 years. The current standard for radiation delivery to thymic tumors is conformal radiotherapy using three-dimensional treatment planning and high-energy (>10 MeV) photons generated by linear accelerators.[2,13] Preliminary steps are (1) the three-dimensional acquisition of anatomic data and (2) computed modelization and treatment planning.[13] A "dosimetric" CT scan is performed in the position of radiotherapy in blocked inspiration, with serial 5-mm cuts and without contrast injection. To ensure a perfect reproducibility along

Disclosure: The authors have no conflict of interest to disclose.
a Radiotherapy Department, Lyon-Sud Hospital, 165 Chemin du Grand Revoyet, F-69495, Pierre-Bénite, France
b Department of Respiratory Medicine, Pilot Unit for the Management of Rare Intrathoracic Tumors, Louis Pradel Hospital, 28 Avenue Doyen Lépine, Lyon 69677, France
c Claude Bernard University, 28 Avenue Rockefeller, Lyon 69008, France
* Corresponding author. Département de Radiothérapie Oncologie, Centre Hospitalier Lyon Sud, 165, Chemin du Grand Revoyet, 69495 Pierre-Bénite Cedex, France.
E-mail address: francoise.mornex@chu-lyon.fr

Thorac Surg Clin 21 (2011) 99–105
doi:10.1016/j.thorsurg.2010.08.011

the planning and treatment procedures, a personalized frame is cast for each patient. The tumor (gross tumor volume [GTV]), and all intrathoracic organs (lung, heart, spinal cord, esophagus, phrenic nerve) are then delineated on each CT scan image. Delineation may be difficult in case of lobar atelectasia secondary to bronchial obstruction or pleural mass. Integration or fusion with data from F18-fluorodeoxyglucose positron emission tomography scan or from MRI may then be useful, but these techniques have not been specifically evaluated for thymic tumors. The delineation leads to the establishment of a personalized three-dimensional virtual model of intrathoracic tumoral and nontumoral structures.

Volumes

Volumes are defined based on pre- and postoperative imaging, with the help of surgical clips placed during the operation. In addition to GTV, which includes the visible extent and location of the tumor, the radiotherapist defines (1) a clinical target volume that encompasses surrounding subclinical microscopic malignant disease by adding a 5 to 7 mm margin around the GTV, and (2) the final planning target volume, with an additional margin for body movements (internal target volume [ITV]) and technical deviations during the treatment course. ITV margins, in the absence of respiratory control, are usually 10 mm for the tumor and 5 mm for lymph nodes. Similarly, the repositioning variation along treatment courses is estimated to be 6 mm on average, with errors higher than 10 mm in 32% of the patients, for an estimated loss of tumor control of 5%. Overall, margins around the GTV usually range from 15 to 25 mm in the absence of respiratory gating, and 10 to 15 mm with respiratory gating (see later discussion). Depending on surgical staging, all areas suspicious of microscopic disease, including the pericardium, great vessels, lung, and regional lymph nodes, are included in the GTV.[14-16] Prophylactic extensive-field irradiation of mediastinal and supraclavicular nodes or of the whole hemithorax is controversial, and is not performed in a routine practice setting. In a series of 169 patients, extended field arrangement did not confer any additional local control benefit, and produced significantly higher lung toxicity rates.[17]

The actual treatment planning step consists of working on the virtual three-dimensional model to determine the number, incidence, and energy of each radiation beam, and the shape of the fields, modeled by personalized masks or a multiblade collimator. Homogeneity correction is integrated in treatment planning, to integrate transmission differentials within the lung parenchyma.[15] The quantification of radiation dose distribution within the virtual model allows several treatment plannings to be compared using dose–volume histograms, which represent for each structure the volume receiving at least a certain radiation dose[15] and normal tissue complication probabilities, which are available for each critical organ.

Doses

Numerous radiation dose and fractionation schemes have been reported for thymoma and thymic carcinomas.[14,16-23] Although thymomas have been recognized as highly radiosensitive tumors for years, the benefit of dose escalation on local control has not clearly been established. Arriagada and colleagues[24] reported similar local control rates with total doses inferior to 48 Gy or superior to 60 Gy. In this series, the local recurrence rate in resected stage III and IV tumors was 80% after adjuvant radiotherapy delivered to median doses of 45 to 50 Gy. Zhu and colleagues[17] reported no difference in local control with doses of 50 Gy or higher than 60 Gy.

The major objective of radiotherapy planning is to deliver to the thymic area a total dose of 45 Gy in a neoadjuvant setting, 45 to 55 Gy in an adjuvant setting, and 60 to 66 Gy as an exclusive treatment,[2,8-11,25] using a standard fractionation scheme (one 1.8- to 2-Gy fraction per day) and without risking severe toxicities on nontumoral tissues. The lung V_{20} (percentage of pulmonary volume receiving at least 20 Gy) must be lower than 35% and the lung V_{30} (percentage of pulmonary volume receiving at least 30 Gy) lower than 20% (and even less in case of chronic obstructive pulmonary disease). Similarly, the maximum dose delivered to the cardiac tissue is 40 Gy, with a cardiac V_{20} lower than 60%. The maximum dose to the spine is 40 Gy per segment. Finally, the volume of esophageal tissue must be limited as much as possible.

Technically, treatment port arrangements historically included a single anterior port, unequally weighted (2:1 or 3:2), or two opposed anterior–posterior fields.[20-23,25] Recently, conformal techniques make multifield arrangement the standard technique.

Radiation Delivery Optimization

Recent technical improvements in the delivery of radiation doses may help optimize radiotherapy for thymic tumors. Intensity modulated radiotherapy (IMRT) consists of a real-time modeling of the contours and the amount of photons delivered within the radiation beam, using a programmed movement of the blades of the collimator.[13] This functionality allows beams of variable shapes to be administered during a single sequence, possibly proving to be helpful to target tumors that are close to critical tissues. This technique has not been specifically evaluated in thymic tumors, but data obtained in lung cancer are promising to reduce lung and heart toxicity rates.[26] In thymic tumors, IMRT may be of great interest in delivering high dose-gradients on pleural recurrences and on lesions abutting the spinal cord. The use of IMRT should then be encouraged and developed in a routine practice setting.

Standard radiotherapy delivers radiation under shallow breathing, and then sufficient ITV must be added so that the prescription dose is reached everywhere within the moving tumor. With so called four-dimensional (4D) techniques, the motion-encompassing volume is much smaller. *Respiratory control* involves assisted or voluntary blocking of respiration in a selected phase of the respiratory cycle, during which radiation is delivered.[13] *Respiratory gating* enables the photon beam only when the motion amplitude coincides with a preselected sector of the respiratory cycle. *Respiratory tracking* involves intentionally moving the irradiating beam so that it follows the movement of the tumor. Again, 4D techniques have not been specifically reported for the treatment of thymic malignancies. Data are lacking regarding mediastinal structures motion from one radiotherapy fraction to another, and therefore evaluating the potential role of 4D techniques in this setting is difficult.

ADJUVANT RADIOTHERAPY FOR RESECTABLE THYMOMA

The role of radiation therapy in the management of early-stage thymoma remains highly debated. The low number and the delay of recurrences cause statistical analyses to be underpowered in most studies. Given the highly significant prognostic value of tumor stage and completeness of surgical resection, the relative weight of radiotherapy in overall survival is hard to evaluate.[5,27]

Masaoka Stage I Thymoma

Masaoka stage I thymomas have a recurrence rate as low as 0.9% to 2% after R0 resection, with a 5-year survival of 100%.[5,20,28–31] Tumor size or presence of pleural adherences do not seem to change these figures.[30] Adjuvant treatment is then unlikely to show any significant improvement. A Chinese trial involving 29 patients compared adjuvant radiotherapy with exclusive surgery in patients with completely resected stage I thymomas, and failed to show any survival difference between the groups.[32] Moreover, tumor recurrences may be eligible for surgical re-resection, which produces similar results to initial treatment.[33] A report from the Survival, Epidemiology and End Results (SEER) database involving 275 stage I thymic tumors suggested a possible adverse impact of postoperative radiotherapy on 5-year cause-specific survival (91% vs 98% without radiotherapy; $P = .03$).[34] Adjuvant radiotherapy is therefore not recommended in stage I thymomas after complete surgical resection.

Masaoka Stage II through III Thymomas

The standard treatment of Masaoka stage II–III resectable thymomas is upfront surgery. For stage II tumors, complete resection is achieved in 75% to 90% of cases, with 5- and 10-year survival rates ranging from 85% to 93%.[5,6,17,20,29,34–37] Given these results, the indications of radiotherapy are highly debated. The Japanese cohort reported by Kondo included 257 stage II thymomas, and no significant difference was observed regarding recurrence rates in patients who underwent surgery alone or surgery followed by adjuvant radiotherapy.[5] However, more recent series suggested that adjuvant radiotherapy might improve disease-free and overall survival even more for these patients; up to 100% and 95%, respectively.[17,30,38,39] However, these data were collected through noncontrolled retrospective design, and therefore are difficult to interpret.

In completely resected Masaoka stage III thymomas, the rationale for adjuvant radiotherapy to reduce local recurrence rates is better established.[18,21,31,40] In a series of 112 patients with invasive thymomas, Curran and colleagues[18] reported that postoperative radiotherapy decreased mediastinal recurrence rate from 53% to 0% in completely resected tumors, and to 21% after incomplete resection. Other studies reported similar figures, with local relapses observed in 0% to 20% and 50% to 60% of cases after surgery followed by adjuvant radiotherapy, or exclusive surgery, respectively.[41–45]

Two large analyses were recently reported that tapered the systematic recommendation of adjuvant radiotherapy in stage II–III thymomas. The SEER analysis included 626 invasive thymic tumors and showed a similar cause-specific survival between patients who underwent adjuvant radiotherapy or those who did not (91% vs 86%; $P = .12$).[34] This finding may be related to the high late toxicity rates after radiotherapy before the conformal era. Moreover, no benefit from radiotherapy was observed after "extirpative" (ie, R0 or R1) resection. Despite intrinsic limitations, this analysis suggests a limited role of adjuvant radiotherapy, especially for stage II tumors with a spontaneously low recurrence rate.

The second study was a meta-analysis of series comparing exclusive surgery versus surgery followed by radiotherapy for stage II–III thymomas, published from 1981 to 2008.[12] This study was actually a pooled analysis of retrospective data, because no prospective trial has been conducted in the field. Overall, 592 patients from 13 studies were included: 250 who received adjuvant radiotherapy, and 342 who did not. No significant difference was observed between the groups (odds ratio, 1.05; $P = .63$; 95% CI, 0.63–1.75).[12] Therefore, adjuvant radiotherapy is highly controversial for invasive thymoma, especially stage II tumors. Integration of other prognostic predictors, such as histology (type B3 vs others[35,36]), tumor size,[35] margins size, and capsular invasion (minimal or extensive), may be useful in identifying patients benefiting from postoperative treatment.

Hemithoracic Radiotherapy

Recurrence after surgery for invasive thymoma mostly occurs in the pleura. Radiotherapy delivered to the thymic area fails to control recurrent pleural dissemination.[46] Several reports indicate the feasibility and efficacy of delivering a 10- to 15-Gy prophylactic hemithoracic irradiation after complete resection and focal adjuvant radiotherapy, a strategy that reduced recurrence rates from 90% to 100% to 60% to 75%.[23,45,47,48] In the retrospective analysis reported by Uematsu and colleagues,[47] 23 patients underwent hemithoracic radiation and 20 patients did not. The first group had higher relapse-free survival (100% vs 74%; $P = .03$) and 5-year survival rates (96% vs 66%; $P = .03$); 13% of patients presented with radiation-induced pneumonitis. In a more recent series, the pleural control was as high as 71% in patients undergoing adjuvant mediastinal radiotherapy and hemithoracic radiation.[49] In this setting, IMRT is a promising technique.

Incomplete Resection

In case of incomplete resection (R1 or R2), adjuvant radiotherapy is systematically recommended to a total dose of 66 Gy, including the boost on areas of macroscopic invasion (ideally marked with surgical clips). Radiotherapy consistently decreased recurrence rates from 60% to 80% to 21% to 45% in this setting.[5,18,20,21,39,44–46]

EXCLUSIVE RADIOTHERAPY

For thymomas definitely judged to be unresectable, radiotherapy or chemoradiation is administered. Only one prospective trial evaluated radiotherapy as a definite treatment for advanced thymoma.[50] Mean total dose was 46 Gy (which is certainly too low). In the 25 patients recruited, disease-free survival was 81% and overall survival was 72%.[50] Retrospective data in unselected population reported a less-impressive outcome, with disease-free survival ranging from 45% to 50%.[48,51]

In this setting, chemoradiation is delivered sequentially to minimize the risk of cumulative toxicities, given the potential radiosensitization with anthracyclines. Definitive chemoradiation combining the adriamycin, cyclophosphamide, and platin chemotherapy with standard radiation to a total dose of 54 Gy produced an overall response rate of 70% and a 5-year survival of 53%, comparing favorably with the results of incomplete resection.[51] Ciernik and colleagues[41] reported a 5-year survival rate of 87% in a small group of patients with stage III and IV disease who did not undergo resection.

RADIOTHERAPY AND MULTIMODALITY TREATMENT FOR ADVANCED-STAGE THYMIC TUMORS

Neoadjuvant radiotherapy has been used in several small-size cohorts of patients with marginally resectable or unresectable stage III or IV thymic tumors, in a multimodal therapeutic strategy setting. In most studies, radiotherapy was sequentially combined with chemotherapy, and therefore the respective role of each modality is difficult to assess. The main objective of this strategy is to reduce the risk of tumor seeding during surgery[41,52] and to increase the R0 resection rate, especially in case of tumor invasion of critical organs.[40,53] Preoperative radiation is more effective on type B1 than on B3 thymomas, with a marked effect on lymphocytes.[54] Response rates up to 80% have been reported for neoadjuvant treatment in highly selected cases. Complete resection may then be achieved in 60% to 75% of cases, far higher than the 50% usually reported in stage III thymomas.[18,52,53,55] Again, the survival impact is difficult to assess. The role of neoadjuvant radiation therapy remains controversial.

Neoadjuvant chemotherapy may provide an observation period to evaluate tumor chemosensitivity before opting for surgery or definitive radiotherapy, which is then delivered to a final total dose of 60 to 66 Gy. In operated cases, adjuvant radiotherapy is usually delivered.[56,57] In the study reported by Wright and colleagues,[58] platin–etoposide combination plus concurrent radiotherapy (total doses ranging from 33 to 49 Gy) produced a 100% disease control rate (40% response rate and 60% stable disease rate).

RADIOTHERAPY AND RECURRENCES

Recurrences of thymoma are usually eligible for surgery.[33] Complete resection may be achieved in 45% to 70% of cases.[33,45] Complete resection is also the most significant prognostic indicator in this setting. In unresectable local recurrences, exclusive radiotherapy may be useful. High response rates, with 5-year survival rates of 70% to 80%, were obtained in small retrospective series.[45] Hemithoracic radiotherapy must be further evaluated in this setting.[49]

RADIOTHERAPY FOR THYMIC CARCINOMA

The optimal treatment of thymic carcinoma remains unclear given the rarity of the tumor.[16] As most thymic carcinoma present with invasive pattern at diagnosis, neoadjuvant chemoradiotherapy may represent a potent approach to downstage unresectable lesions.[28,59] The effect of radiotherapy on disease-free and overall survival in patients with thymic carcinoma is expected to be higher than that of patients with thymoma given the lower importance of surgery. However, for the 186 cases of thymic carcinoma reported in the Kondo study, 5-year survival rates after complete resection were 74% after adjuvant radiotherapy and 72% without adjuvant radiotherapy.[5] More recent series systematically reported the use of postoperative radiotherapy.[28,59–61] Doses ranged from 40 to 70 Gy with standard fractionation scheme (1.8–2.0 Gy per fraction). In a series of 26 patients treated with surgery and postoperative radiation without chemotherapy, survival was as high as 77%, with 82% and 66% survival rates after R0 and R1 resection, respectively.[28]

RADIOTHERAPY TOXICITIES

The side effects of radiation are linked to the type and volume of tissue treated, and to the dose administered during in each treatment session and the whole treatment.[13] Individual factors, including genetic susceptibility, may also participate in the prediction of toxicity. Thoracic radiotherapy may produce major toxicities in the heart, the spinal cord, the lung, and the esophagus. Most frequent acute symptoms include transient esophagitis, pericarditis, and pneumonitis. Late toxicities are even more crucial to consider for thymic tumors given the prolonged survival of patients, contrary to more frequent thoracic malignancies such as lung cancer. These effects are not systematically recorded given loss of follow-up issues. Major radiation-induced late toxicities are pulmonary fibrosis and cardiac diseases (pericarditis, coronary abnormalities, congestive heart failure, cardiomyopathy). The use of anthracycline-based chemotherapy makes dose delivered to the heart a major constraint for treatment planning.[15] Earlier reports estimated grade 3 to 4 toxicities occurred in 10–15% of patients.[21,41,45] Radiation-related deaths occur in fewer than 1% of cases in modern series.[13,15]

SUMMARY

Radiotherapy is a major therapeutic modality for thymic malignancies. The exact role of adjuvant radiotherapy after complete resection is still debated for stage II–III tumors. Histology or size, capsular invasion, and even molecular data[62] may be included in the decision making. Radiotherapy may be recommended for stage III thymomas, thymic carcinoma, or after incomplete surgical resection. Combination with chemotherapy may be useful, and must be further evaluated using validated end points, including 5- and 10-year time-to-progression and overall survival. Several initiatives have been taken worldwide to launch collaborative studies in the field,[63] including prospective trials specifically readdressing the role of radiotherapy for thymic malignancies.

REFERENCES

1. de Jong WK, Blaauwgeers JL, Schaapveld M, et al. Thymic epithelial tumours: a population-based study of the incidence, diagnostic procedures and therapy. Eur J Cancer 2008;44(1):123–30.
2. Girard N, Mornex F, Van Houtte P, et al. Thymoma: a focus on current therapeutic management. J Thorac Oncol 2009;4(1):119–26.
3. WHO histological classification of tumours of the thymus. In: Travis WB, Brambilla A, Muller-Hermelinck HK, et al, editors. World Health Organization classification of tumours. Pathology and genetics of tumours of the lung, pleura, thymus and heart. Lyon (France): IARC Press; 2004. p. 146.
4. Masaoka A, Monden Y, Nakahara K, et al. Follow-up study of thymomas with special reference to their clinical stages. Cancer 1981;48(11):2485–92.
5. Kondo K, Monden Y. Therapy for thymic epithelial tumors: a clinical study of 1,320 patients from Japan. Ann Thorac Surg 2003;76(3):878–84.

6. Blumberg D, Port JL, Weksler B, et al. Thymoma: a multivariate analysis of factors predicting survival. Ann Thorac Surg 1995;60(4):908–13.

7. Eng TY, Fuller CD, Jagirdar J, et al. Thymic carcinoma: state of the art review. Int J Radiat Oncol Biol Phys 2004;59(3):654–64.

8. Tomaszek S, Wigle DA, Keshavjee S, et al. Thymomas: review of current clinical practice. Ann Thorac Surg 2009;87(6):1973–80.

9. Kong FM, Lu JJ. Thymoma. In: Brady LW, Lu JJ, Heilmann HP, et al, editors. Radiation oncology: an evidence-based approach. Berlin, Heidelberg: Springer-Verlag; 2008. p. 159–70.

10. Falkson CB, Bezjak A, Darling G, et al. The management of thymoma: a systematic review and practice guideline. J Thorac Oncol 2009;4(7):911–9.

11. NCCN Clinical Practice Guidelines in Oncology. Thymic malignancies. V.2.2010. Available at: www.nccn.org. Accessed September 18, 2010.

12. Korst RJ, Kansler AL, Christos PJ, et al. Adjuvant radiotherapy for thymic epithelial tumors: a systematic review and meta-analysis. Ann Thorac Surg 2009;87(5):1641–7.

13. Girard N, Mornex F. Radiotherapy for locally advanced non-small cell lung cancer. Eur J Cancer 2009;45S1:113–25.

14. Fuller CD, Housman DM, Thomas CR. Radiotherapy for thymoma and thymic carcinoma. Hematol Oncol Clin North Am 2008;22(3):489–507.

15. Moiseenko V, Craig T, Bezjak A, et al. Dose-volume analysis of lung complications in the radiation treatment of malignant thymoma: a retrospective review. Radiother Oncol 2003;67(3):265–74.

16. Eng TY, Thomas CR Jr. Radiation therapy in the management of thymic tumors. Semin Thorac Cardiovasc Surg 2005;17(1):32–40.

17. Zhu G, He S, Fu X, et al. Radiotherapy and prognostic factors for thymoma: a retrospective study of 175 patients. Int J Radiat Oncol Biol Phys 2004; 60(4):1113–9.

18. Curran WJ Jr, Kornstein MJ, Brooks JJ, et al. Invasive thymoma: the role of mediastinal irradiation following complete or incomplete surgical resection. J Clin Oncol 1988;6(11):1722–7.

19. Arakawa A, Yasunaga T, Saitoh Y, et al. Radiation therapy of invasive thymoma. Int J Radiat Oncol Biol Phys 1990;18(3):529–34.

20. Cowen D, Richaud P, Mornex F, et al. Thymoma: results of a multicentric retrospective series of 149 non-metastatic irradiated patients and review of the literature. FNCLCC trialists. Fédération Nationale des Centres de Lutte Contre le Cancer. Radiother Oncol 1995;34(1):9–16.

21. Mornex F, Resbeut M, Richaud P, et al. Radiotherapy and chemotherapy for invasive thymomas: a multicentric retrospective review of 90 cases. The FNCLCC trialists. Fédération Nationale des Centres de Lutte Contre le Cancer. Int J Radiat Oncol Biol Phys 1995;32(3):651–9.

22. Latz D, Schraube P, Oppitz U, et al. Invasive thymoma: treatment with postoperative radiation therapy. Radiology 1997;204(3):859–64.

23. Haniuda M, Miyazawa M, Yoshida K, et al. Is postoperative radiotherapy for thymoma effective? Ann Surg 1996;224(2):219–24.

24. Arriagada R, Gerard-Marchant R, Tubiana M, et al. Radiation therapy in the management of malignant thymic tumors. Acta Radiol Oncol 1981;20(3): 167–72.

25. Park HS, Shin DM, Lee JS, et al. Thymoma. A retrospective study of 87 cases. Cancer 1994;73(10): 2491–8.

26. Chapet O, Khodri M, Jalade P, et al. Potential benefits of using non coplanar field and intensity modulated radiation therapy to preserve the heart in irradiation of lung tumors in the middle and lower lobes. Radiother Oncol 2006;80(3):333–40.

27. Rossi G, Costantini M, Tagliavini E, et al. Thymoma classification: does it matter. Histopathology 2008; 53(4):483–4.

28. Hsu HC, Huang EY, Wang CJ, et al. Postoperative radiotherapy in thymic carcinoma: treatment results and prognostic factors. Int J Radiat Oncol Biol Phys 2002;52(3):801–5.

29. Utsumi T, Shiono H, Kadota Y, et al. Postoperative radiation therapy after complete resection of thymoma has little impact on survival. Cancer 2009;115(23): 5413–20.

30. Wu KL, Mao JF, Chen GY, et al. Prognostic predictors and long-term outcome of postoperative irradiation in thymoma: a study of 241 patients. Cancer Invest 2009;27(10):1008–15.

31. Singhal S, Shrager JB, Rosenthal DI, et al. Comparison of stages I–II thymoma treated by complete resection with or without adjuvant radiation. Ann Thorac Surg 2003;76(5):1635–41.

32. Zhang H, Lu N, Wang M, et al. Postoperative radiotherapy for stage I thymoma: a prospective randomized trial in 29 cases. Chin Med J (Engl) 1999; 112(2):136–8.

33. Lucchi M, Basolo F, Mussi A. Surgical treatment of pleural recurrence from thymoma. Eur J Cardiothorac Surg 2008;33(4):707–11.

34. Forquer JA, Rong N, Fakiris AJ, et al. Postoperative radiotherapy after surgical resection of thymoma: differing roles in localized and regional disease. Int J Radiat Oncol Biol Phys 2010;76(2): 440–5.

35. Chen YD, Feng QF, Lu HZ, et al. Role of adjuvant radiotherapy for stage II thymoma after complete tumor resection. Int J Radiat Oncol Biol Phys 2010. [Epub ahead of print].

36. Ogawa K, Uno T, Toita T, et al. Postoperative radiotherapy for patients with completely resected

thymoma: a multi-institutional, retrospective review of 103 patients. Cancer 2002;94(5):1405–13.

37. Wilkins KB, Sheikh E, Green R, et al. Clinical and pathologic predictors of survival in patients with thymoma. Ann Surg 1999;230(4):562–72.

38. Kundel Y, Yellin A, Popovtzer A, et al. Adjuvant radiotherapy for thymic epithelial tumor: treatment results and prognostic factors. Am J Clin Oncol 2007;30(4): 389–94.

39. Mangi AA, Wright CD, Allan JS, et al. Adjuvant radiation therapy for stage II thymoma. Ann Thorac Surg 2002;74(4):1033–7.

40. Myojin M, Choi NC, Wright CD, et al. Stage III thymoma: pattern of failure after surgery and postoperative radiotherapy and its implication for future study. Int J Radiat Oncol Biol Phys 2000;46(4): 927–33.

41. Ciernik IF, Meier U, Lütolf UM. Prognostic factors and outcome of incompletely resected invasive thymoma following radiation therapy. J Clin Oncol 1994; 12(7):1484–90.

42. Nakahara K, Ohno K, Hashimoto J, et al. Thymoma: results with complete resection and adjuvant postoperative irradiation in 141 consecutive patients. J Thorac Cardiovasc Surg 1988;95(6):1041–7.

43. Haniuda M, Morimoto M, Nishimura H, et al. Adjuvant radiotherapy after complete resection of thymoma. Ann Thorac Surg 1992;54(2):311–5.

44. Pollack A, Komaki R, Cox JD, et al. Thymoma: treatment and prognosis. Int J Radiat Oncol Biol Phys 1992;23(5):1037–43.

45. Urgesi A, Monetti U, Rossi G, et al. Aggressive treatment of intrathoracic recurrences of thymoma. Radiother Oncol 1992;24(4):221–5.

46. Jackson MA, Ball DL. Post-operative radiotherapy in invasive thymoma. Radiother Oncol 1991;21(2): 77–82.

47. Uematsu M, Yoshida H, Kondo M, et al. Entire hemithorax irradiation following complete resection in patients with stage II–III invasive thymoma. Int J Radiat Oncol Biol Phys 1996;35(2):357–60.

48. Yoshida H, Uematsu M, Itami J, et al. The role of low-dose hemithoracic radiotherapy for thoracic dissemination of thymoma. Radiat Med 1997;15(6): 399–403.

49. Sugie C, Shibamoto Y, Ikeya-Hashizume C, et al. Invasive thymoma: postoperative mediastinal irradiation, and low-dose entire hemithorax irradiation in patients with pleural dissemination. J Thorac Oncol 2008;3(1):75–81.

50. Sur RK, Pacella JA, Donde B, et al. Role of radiotherapy in stage III invasive thymomas. S Afr J Surg 1997;35(4):206–9.

51. Loehrer, Sr PJ, Chen M, Kim K, et al. Cisplatin, doxorubicin, and cyclophosphamide plus thoracic radiation therapy for limited-stage unresectable thymoma: an intergroup trial. J Clin Oncol 1997; 15(9):3093–9.

52. Ohara K, Okumura T, Sugahara S, et al. The role of preoperative radiotherapy for invasive thymoma. Acta Oncol 1990;29(4):425–9.

53. Akaogi E, Ohara K, Mitsui K, et al. Preoperative radiotherapy and surgery for advanced thymoma with invasion to the great vessels. J Surg Oncol 1996;63(1):17–22.

54. Onuki T, Ishikawa S, Yamamoto T, et al. Pathologic radioresponse of preoperatively irradiated invasive thymomas. J Thorac Oncol 2008;3(3):270–6.

55. Okumura M, Miyoshi S, Takeuchi Y, et al. Results of surgical treatment of thymomas with special reference to the involved organs. J Thorac Cardiovasc Surg 1999;117(3):605–13.

56. Shin DM, Walsh GL, Komaki R, et al. A multidisciplinary approach to therapy for unresectable malignant thymoma. Ann Intern Med 1998; 129(2):100–4.

57. Venuta F, Rendina EA, Pescarmona EO, et al. Multimodality treatment of thymoma: a prospective study. Ann Thorac Surg 1997;64(6):1585–91.

58. Wright CD, Choi NC, Wain JC, et al. Induction chemoradiotherapy followed by resection for locally advanced Masaoka stage III and IVA thymic tumors. Ann Thorac Surg 2008;85(2):385–9.

59. Magois E, Guigay J, Blancard PS, et al. Multimodal treatment of thymic carcinoma: report of nine cases. Lung Cancer 2008;59(1):126–32.

60. Ogawa K, Toita T, Uno T, et al. Treatment and prognosis of thymic carcinoma: a retrospective analysis of 40 cases. Cancer 2002;94(12):3115–9.

61. Takeda S, Sawabata N, Inoue M, et al. Thymic carcinoma. Clinical institutional experience with 15 patients. Eur J Cardiothorac Surg 2004;26(2): 401–6.

62. Girard N, Shen R, Guo T, et al. Comprehensive genomic analysis reveals clinically relevant molecular distinctions between thymic carcinomas and thymomas. Clin Cancer Res 2009;15(22):6790–9.

63. Detterbeck F, Giaccone G, Loehrer P, et al. International thymic malignancy interest group. J Thorac Oncol 2010;5(1):1–2.

Chemotherapy for Thymic Tumors: Induction, Consolidation, Palliation

Arun Rajan, MD, Giuseppe Giaccone, MD, PhD*

KEYWORDS

• Thymoma • Thymic carcinoma • Chemotherapy

Thymoma and thymic carcinoma are rare tumors with a spectrum of biologic behavior that ranges from relatively indolent to highly aggressive. Systemic chemotherapy is primarily used in patients who present with unresectable or recurrent disease. Responses to a number of different chemotherapeutic agents have been documented in the literature; however, given the rarity of these tumors, there is a paucity of data from prospective trials. Well-evaluated regimens consist of a combination of drugs that almost always include a platinum compound. In recent years, high-dose chemotherapy has also been evaluated for the treatment of thymic malignancies. Based on the intent of treatment, chemotherapy can be administered in the neoadjuvant setting or for palliation of advanced disease.

INDUCTION CHEMOTHERAPY

Surgery plays a key role in the successful management of thymic malignancies. Because these tumors are responsive to chemotherapy and radiation, attempts have been made to incorporate these modalities before and after surgery to improve survival and decrease the chance of recurrence. Induction chemotherapy and chemoradiotherapy are used to decrease the size of tumors before surgery so as to make potentially unresectable tumors resectable and increase the

chance of having a complete resection. Complete resection is in fact one of the most important prognostic factors together with stage and histologic type in thymic malignancies.[1]

Wright and colleagues[2] performed a retrospective review of a series of 10 patients with stage III and IVA thymic tumors (9 thymomas and 1 thymic carcinoma) who were treated with induction chemoradiotherapy followed by resection and then adjuvant chemotherapy. Patients were deemed to have unresectable disease at the outset. Chemotherapy consisted of cisplatin 33 mg/m^2 daily ×3 plus etoposide 100 mg/m^2 daily ×3. Two cycles were planned 3 to 4 weeks apart. Concurrent radiation therapy was delivered with a target dose of 40 to 45 Gy. Surgical resection was then performed with a goal of complete resection. Postoperative chemotherapy with cisplatin and etoposide was planned for patients with incomplete resections and those judged to be at high risk for recurrence. Of 10 patients treated with chemoradiotherapy, 40% had a partial response (PR) and 60% had stable disease (SD). Eight patients went on to have a complete resection (R0 resection) and 2 patients had a microscopically incomplete resection (R1 resection). Two patients had a near-complete pathologic response with greater than 99% necrosis and 2 patients had microscopic residual disease with greater than 90% necrosis. Seven patients received postoperative chemotherapy. Two patients had

Medical Oncology Branch, National Cancer Institute, National Institutes of Health, 10 Center Drive, Building 10, Room 12N226, Bethesda, MD 20892, USA

* Corresponding author.

E-mail address: giacconeg@mail.nih.gov

Thorac Surg Clin 21 (2011) 107–114

doi:10.1016/j.thorsurg.2010.08.003

1547-4127/11/$ — see front matter. Published by Elsevier Inc.

complications after surgery including one case of tamponade after pleuropneumonectomy with pericardial resection and another case of acute respiratory distress syndrome in a patient who had low-grade treatment-related pneumonitis after induction therapy. There were no postoperative deaths. After a median follow-up of 41 months, 3 patients had disease recurrence. The estimated 5-year survival was 69% (95% confidence interval [CI], 32% to 100%).

Ishikawa and colleagues[3] reported results from a series of 11 patients with stage IV thymoma (7 World Health Organization [WHO] B2 subtype, 3 WHO B3, 1 WHO B3+C) and pleural dissemination treated with multimodality therapy consisting of induction chemotherapy followed by thymectomy and postoperative therapy (adjuvant radiation therapy in 6 patients and adjuvant chemotherapy in 4 patients). Induction chemotherapy consisted of cisplatin, doxorubicin, and methylprednisolone (CAMP) in 7 patients, and cisplatin, doxorubicin, cyclophosphamide, and etoposide (PACE) in 1 patient. Six patients had a PR and 2 patients had SD for an objective response rate of 75%. The response rate to CAMP therapy was 85%. Surgical resection was then performed in 10 patients. There were no surgery-related deaths. Overall survival with multimodality treatment was 81% at 5 years and 70% at 10 years.

Yokoi and colleagues[4] used the CAMP induction therapy as part of a multimodality regimen in patients with advanced thymoma. The CAMP regimen consisted of cisplatin 20 mg/m^2/day intravenously (IV) from days 1 to 4, doxorubicin 40 mg/m^2 IV on day 1, and methylprednisolone 1000 mg/day IV on days 1 to 4 and 500 mg/day IV on days 5 and 6. Treatment was repeated every 21 to 28 days. Seventeen patients were enrolled in this study including 4 patients with stage III, 9 with stage IVA, and 4 with stage IVB disease. In 14 of 17 patients who received CAMP chemotherapy, an overall response rate of 93% (95% CI, 66.1%– 99.8%) was noted including 1 complete response (CR) and 13 PRs. The most frequent grade 3/4 adverse events were leucopenia and neutropenia. There was one chemotherapy-related death. Nine patients underwent surgery and 8 patients went on to receive postoperative radiation therapy. The 5-year overall survival (OS) rate for all 17 patients in this trial was 81%.

A prospective analysis of 30 patients with stage III–IVA thymomas who underwent neoadjuvant chemotherapy, surgery, and adjuvant therapy was reported by Lucchi and colleagues.[5] Neoadjuvant therapy consisted of cisplatin 75 mg/m^2 on day 1; epirubicin 100 mg/m^2 on day 1; and etoposide 120 mg/m^2 on days 1, 3, and 5 of a 3-week cycle. Three cycles of chemotherapy were administered followed by a restaging to evaluate for response. A total of 89 cycles of neoadjuvant chemotherapy were administered. Two CRs (7%), 20 PRs (67%), and 8 SD (27%) were seen. Neutropenic fever was seen with 23 courses (26%) of therapy. No grade 4 nonhematological toxicity was noted and grade 3 nonhematological toxicity included alopecia with 21 cycles of therapy and nausea/emesis with 1 cycle. Surgery was performed in all 30 patients; resection was complete in 23 cases and incomplete in 7 cases. There was no postoperative mortality. Adjuvant therapy consisted of radiation therapy in 21 patients, chemoradiotherapy in 8 patients, and chemotherapy in 1 patient. Ten-year survival was 86% with stage III disease and 76% with stage IVA disease. The investigators concluded that the high response rate to neoadjuvant chemotherapy helped in increasing the rate of complete resection in this patient population.

Bretti and colleagues[6] published results from a series of 63 consecutive patients with malignant thymoma treated with a multimodal approach. Forty-three patients had stage III disease and 20 patients had stage IVA disease. Thirty-three patients were not considered candidates for radical surgery as the initial treatment. Among these patients, preoperative radiation therapy was administered in 8 patients and neoadjuvant chemotherapy was administered in 25 patients (40%). Eighteen patients received the ADOC regimen consisting of doxorubicin 40 mg/m^2 and cisplatin 50 mg/m^2 on day 1, vincristine 0.6 mg/m^2 on day 2, and cyclophosphamide 700 mg/m^2 on day 4, every 3 weeks. Seven patients received a combination of cisplatin 100 mg/m^2 on day 1 and etoposide 100 mg/m^2 on days 1 to 3 every 3 weeks. A total of 4 cycles of neoadjuvant chemotherapy were planned. Responses included 2 CRs (8%), 16 PRs (64%), 6 SD (24%), and 1 patient with progressive disease (PD) (4%). Among the patients who received neoadjuvant chemotherapy, 14 patients (56%) underwent surgery and complete resection could be performed in 11 cases (44%). There were no deaths related to surgery. Postoperative treatment consisted of radiation therapy. Median progression-free survival (PFS) for patients undergoing radical resection after receiving neoadjuvant therapy was 56.9 months (19.2 months to 94.5 months). In comparison, median PFS had not been reached for patients undergoing radical surgical resection as the initial treatment and it was 11.9 months (95% CI, 0–25.6) for patients who did not undergo complete surgical resection. Median OS had not been reached for those patients who underwent radical resection initially and also in those patients who received neoadjuvant therapy followed by radical resection. In patients with incomplete resection, median OS was 43.9 months (27.8—59.8). Administration of neoadjuvant therapy increased the radical resection rate from 46% to 65% in patients with stage III thymoma and from 0% to 20% in patients with stage IVA disease.

Shin and colleagues[7] conducted a prospective trial to evaluate induction chemotherapy with cisplatin 30 mg/m^2/d on days 1 to 3, doxorubicin 20 mg/m^2/d on days 1 to 3, cyclophosphamide 500 mg/m^2 on day 1, and prednisone 100 mg/d for 5 days administered in 3- to 4-week cycles in patients with newly diagnosed, unresectable stage III or IVA malignant thymoma. Induction therapy was followed by surgical resection and postoperative treatment consisting of radiation therapy and 3 cycles of the same chemotherapy regimen with 80% doses of cisplatin, doxorubicin, and cyclophosphamide and 100% doses of prednisone. Thirteen patients were enrolled and 12 were evaluable for response. Following induction therapy, 3 (25%) patients had a CR, 8 (67%) PR, and 1 (8%) minor response. In 11 patients who underwent surgical resection, an R0 resection was possible in 9 (82%) patients, and an incomplete resection in 2 (18%) patients. After completion of planned therapy, the disease-free survival and overall survival rates at 7 years were 73% and 100% respectively. Common side effects associated with chemotherapy were myelosuppression, fatigue, nausea, emesis, and loss of appetite. There was no mortality related to surgery.

Venuta and colleagues[8] conducted a prospective study of multimodality therapy in 65 patients with thymoma. Twenty-five patients in this series had malignant thymomas including stage III and IV cortical thymomas and stage III mixed thymomas. Also included in this group were 5 patients with limited areas of well-differentiated thymic carcinoma. Those patients in this group who were considered to have highly invasive stage III and stage IV lesions or were not candidates for radical resection as initial therapy underwent neoadjuvant chemotherapy followed by surgical resection and postoperative chemotherapy and radiation therapy. Neoadjuvant chemotherapy consisted of cisplatin 75 mg/m^2 to 100 mg/m^2 on day 1; epirubicin 100 mg/m^2 on day 1; and etoposide 120 mg/m^2 on days 1, 3, and 5, repeated every 3 weeks. Three cycles were delivered before surgery and 2 to 3 cycles postoperatively. Eight of 12 patients with stage III disease received neoadjuvant chemotherapy. One patient had a complete remission and 7 patients showed a radiological

response to therapy. Two patients were downstaged from stage III to stage II. All 13 patients with stage IVA disease underwent neoadjuvant chemotherapy. At the time of surgery there was evidence of residual mediastinal tumor in all patients; however, there was a response at metastatic sites in all patients. The rate of radical resection at the time of surgery was 83.3% (10 of 12) in patients with stage III disease and 76.9% (10 of 13) in patients with stage IVA disease. There was no operative mortality. Treatment was generally well tolerated. Adverse events included myelosuppression, alopecia, stomatitis, nausea, and emesis. The median period of follow-up was 53 months (2 to 101 months). Patients with stage III and IV disease demonstrated improved survival compared with a retrospective series of 83 patients reported previously by the same investigators who had undergone surgery but did not receive any adjuvant therapy.

The Japan Clinical Oncology Group (JCOG) performed a phase II trial of dose-dense chemotherapy before surgery and/or radiation therapy in patients with locally advanced thymoma (JCOG 9606).[9] Patients with unresectable stage III thymoma received 9 weeks of chemotherapy with cisplatin 25 mg/m^2 administered weekly from weeks 1 to 9, vincristine 1 mg/m^2 (weeks 1, 2, 4, 6, and 8), doxorubicin 40 mg/m^2 (weeks 1, 3, 5, 7, and 9), and etoposide 80 mg/m^2 daily for 3 days (week 1, 3, 5, 7, and 9). Patients deemed to have resectable disease went on to have surgery followed by radiation therapy and those patients who had unresectable disease received radiation therapy only. Twenty-three patients were enrolled and 57% completed neoadjuvant chemotherapy as planned. Of 21 patients eligible for response, 13 (62%) had a PR (95% CI, 38%—82%), 7 SD, and 1 PD. Thoracotomy was performed in 13 patients with 9 (39%) patients undergoing a complete resection. Major grade 3/4 toxicities related to chemotherapy included anemia (83%), neutropenia (61%), leucopenia (57%), thrombocytopenia (26%), emesis (13%), and infection (13%). Infection in the setting of neutropenia was seen in 1 case only. There were no deaths related to surgery. Median PFS after multimodality therapy was 4.5 years and PFS at 5 years was 43% (95% CI, 21%—63%). Median OS had not been reached at the time of reporting and OS at 5 years was 85% (95% CI, 61%—95%). The investigators concluded that the activity of dose-dense chemotherapy was similar to that of conventional regimen.

Other regimens used for neoadjuvant therapy of thymic malignancies are outlined in **Table 1**.

Table 1
Chemotherapy regimens used for neoadjuvant therapy of thymic malignancies

References	Chemotherapy	Stage	No. of Patients	Responses (%CR+PR)	Stable Disease	TTP, mo	Median Survival, mo
Macchiarini[10]	Cisplatin, Epirubicin, Etoposide	IIIa	7	7 PR (100%)	0	NR	NR (projected 2-y survival 80%)
Berruti[11]	Doxorubicin Cisplatin Vincristine Cyclophosphamide	III (10) IVA (6)	16	1 CR, 12 PR (81%)	2	33.2	47.5
Kim[12]	Cyclophosphamide Doxorubicin Cisplatin Prednisone	III (11) IVA (10) IVB (1)	22	3 CR, 14 PR (77%)	4	NR (PFS at 5-y 77%)	NR (5-y survival 95%)
Jacot[13]	Cisplatin Doxorubicin Cyclophosphamide	III (3) IV (5)	8	6 PR (75%)	1	NR	NR
Rea[14]	Doxorubicin Cisplatin Vincristine Cyclophosphamide	III IVA	16	7CR, 9PR (100%)	0	NR	66

Abbreviations: CR, complete response; NR, not reported; PFS, progression-free survival; PR, partial response; TTP, time to progression.

PALLIATIVE CHEMOTHERAPY

Patients presenting with advanced disease that is deemed unresectable at the time of presentation are candidates for systemic chemotherapy. Many chemotherapeutic drugs have demonstrated single-agent activity against thymic malignancies. In addition, a number of different platinum-based combinations have been evaluated in the treatment of thymic tumors.

The Eastern Cooperative Oncology Group (ECOG) conducted a phase II trial of cisplatin at a dose of 50 mg/m^2 IV every 3 weeks in patients with advanced/recurrent thymoma.[15] Twenty-four patients were enrolled and 20 were evaluable for response. Two (10%) patients demonstrated a PR, 8 (40%) had SD, and 10 (50%) had PD. Toxicity included severe nausea and emesis in 4 patients. Median survival was 76 weeks and 2-year survival was 39%.

Highley and colleagues[16] treated 15 patients with invasive thymoma with single-agent ifosfamide and mesna using 2 different schedules for 5 consecutive days every 3 weeks. In 13 patients evaluable for response, 5 CRs (39%; 95% CI, 18%–65%) and 1 PR (8%; 95% CI, 1%–33%) were seen. The median duration of complete response was 66+ months (range, 25 to 87 months), and the estimated 5-year survival rate was 57%. Treatment was generally well tolerated with the most frequent toxicities being nausea, emesis, and leucopenia.

Results of a phase II study evaluating the role of pemetrexed in patients with recurrent thymoma and thymic carcinoma were reported in abstract form in 2006.[17] In this trial, 16 patients with recurrent thymoma and 11 patients with thymic carcinoma participated. The median number of prior therapies was 2, and 21 patients had received prior radiation therapy. In 23 evaluable patients, 2 CRs and 2 PRs were noted. All 4 responding patients had stage IVA thymoma. The median time to progression for patients with recurrent thymoma was 45.4 weeks, and in patients with thymic carcinoma it was 5.1 weeks. This study demonstrated the activity of pemetrexed in patients with recurrent thymoma.

Although no prospective studies have been conducted to demonstrate the activity of single-agent taxanes in recurrent thymic malignancies, case reports have been published documenting response to paclitaxel and docetaxel.[18,19]

Chahinian and colleagues[20] reported responses to different chemotherapeutic agents in their series of 11 patients with invasive or metastatic thymoma. Eight patients received systemic chemotherapy. The combination of bleomycin, doxorubicin, cisplatin, and prednisone (BAPP) was administered to 5 patients. Two patients had PRs with the responses lasting for 12 months and 4 months. Three patients had disease stabilization. Adverse events associated with therapy included nausea, emesis, and alopecia.

An Intergroup trial evaluated a combination of cisplatin, doxorubicin, and cyclophosphamide (PAC) in patients with unresectable or advanced stage disease who received up to 8 cycles of PAC.[21] In 30 patients assessable for response, 3 CRs and 12 PRs were observed for an overall response rate (ORR) of 50%. The median time to treatment failure was 18.4 months and median survival was 38 months. Estimated 5-year survival was 32% ± 12%. Treatment was generally well tolerated. Predominantly hematological toxicity was seen including one case of febrile neutropenia. No grade 4 nonhematological toxicity was observed.

A phase II trial was conducted to evaluate combined-modality therapy with PAC and thoracic radiation therapy in patients with limited-stage unresectable thymoma.[22] Twenty-six patients enrolled initially of whom 3 patients were found to be ineligible upon pathology review. Treatment consisted of 2 to 4 cycles of PAC chemotherapy administered every 3 weeks. Patients who achieved an objective response or disease stabilization received definitive radiation therapy to the mediastinum and the involved field. Twenty-three patients were assessable for response and survival including 21 patients with thymoma and 2 patients with thymic carcinoma. Toxicity was primarily hematologic including 3 cases of neutropenic fever. One early death occurred related to a perforated abdominal viscus. Responses included 5 CRs and 11 PRs to initial chemotherapy for an objective response rate of 70% (95% CI, 47% to 87%). One of 11 PRs was converted to a CR after subsequent radiation therapy. Four of 5 patients with disease stabilization after initial chemotherapy had an objective response after receiving radiation therapy. The median time to treatment failure was 93.2 months (range, 3 to 99.2+ months). The Kaplan-Meier estimate of median survival was 93 months (range, 1 to 110 months) and the 5-year survival was calculated to be 52.5%. Combined modality therapy appeared to produce durable responses compared with radiation therapy alone.

The combination of doxorubicin, cisplatin, vincristine, and cyclophosphamide (ADOC) was evaluated by Fornasiero and colleagues.[23] Thirty-seven patients with stage III or IV invasive thymoma were enrolled and treatment was administered every 4 weeks. The overall response rate was 92% including complete remission in 43%

cases. Median duration of response was 12 months (2 to 96 + months) and median survival was 15 months (5 to 96 + months) after a median of 5 cycles of therapy.

The European Organization for Research and Treatment of Cancer Lung Cancer Cooperative Group conducted a phase II study to evaluate a combination of cisplatin and etoposide in 16 patients with recurrent or metastatic stage III/IV thymoma.[24] A median of 6 cycles of therapy was administered. In 15 patients assessable for response, 5 CRs and 4 PRs were seen for an overall response rate of 60% (95% CI, 32% to 84%). The median duration of response was 3.4 years (4 months—78 + months). With a median follow-up time of 7 years, the median PFS was 2.2 years and median survival was 4.3 years. PFS and OS at 5 years was 38% and 50% respectively. Frequent adverse events included nausea, emesis, leucopenia, and alopecia.

Loehrer and colleagues[25] reported results of an Intergroup trial that evaluated a combination of ifosfamide, etoposide, and cisplatin (VIP) in 28 evaluable patients with advanced thymic malignancies including 20 patients with thymoma and 8 patients with thymic carcinoma. Six patients had stage III, 13 had stage IVA, and 9 had stage IVB disease. A median of 4 cycles of therapy was administered (1 to 6 cycles). No CRs and 9 PRs were observed, yielding an objective response rate of 32% (95% CI, 16% to 52%). The median duration of response was 12 months (<1 to 26 months). Median survival was 32 months with 2-year survival of 70% estimated by the Kaplan-Meier method. Grade 3/4 toxicity was mainly hematological in 34 patients evaluable for toxicity including thrombocytopenia (53%), leucopenia (47%), and neutropenia (18%).

A phase II study was conducted to assess the anti-tumor activity of interleukin-2 (IL-2) in patients with thymoma.[26] Fourteen patients who had received prior chemotherapy were enrolled and treated with IL-2 at a dose of 12 million units/m^2/d for 5 days weekly for 4 weeks of a 6-week cycle. In the absence of disease progression, a maximum of 4 cycles of treatment were administered. No objective responses were seen with this regimen. Toxicities included anorexia, nausea, hyperbilirubinemia, elevated alanine aminotransferase (ALT), and skin desquamation. Two patients developed new symptoms of myasthenia gravis while on study.

Igawa and colleagues[27] reported results of a retrospective analysis of a series of 11 patients with thymic carcinoma treated with carboplatin and paclitaxel in the first-line setting. The median age was 54 years (32—67) and histologic subtypes included: squamous cell carcinoma (4), large cell neuroendocrine carcinoma (3), small cell carcinoma (1), basaloid subtype (1) and unclassified thymic carcinoma (2). Patients received paclitaxel at a dose of 200 mg/m^2 followed by carboplatin at an AUC of 6 on day 1 of a three week cycle. The median number of cycles administered was 4 (2—6). Four PRs, 5 SD, and 2 PD were seen for an overall response rate of 36% (95% CI, 2.4%—70%). Median PFS was 7.9 months (95% CI, 4—11.7 months) and median OS was 22.7 months (95% CI, 13.3—32.1 months). Median PFS and OS were longer in patients with squamous cell carcinoma compared with non-squamous cell carcinoma (18.8 mo vs 6.9 mo and >31 mo vs 16.3 mo respectively). Major grade 3/4 adverse events included leucopenia (45%), neutropenia (82%), and anemia (18%).

E1C99 was a phase II study of carboplatin and paclitaxel in advanced thymoma and thymic carcinoma. Forty-six patients with unresectable thymoma and thymic carcinoma were enrolled and treated with carboplatin (AUC5) and paclitaxel (225 mg/m^2) on day 1 of a 3-week cycle for a maximum of 6 cycles of therapy. Three CRs and 5 PRs were observed in 24 patients with thymoma for an overall response rate of 33% (90% CI, 18%—52%). No CR and 5 PRs were observed in 21 patients with thymic carcinoma for a response rate of 24% (90% CI, 10%—44%). PFS for the 2 groups was 19.8 months and 6.2 months respectively. Median survival time was 15 months for patients with thymic carcinoma but had not been reached for patients with thymoma when results of this study were reported in 2008. The most common serious adverse event was neutropenia that was seen in 13 (28%) of 46 patients.

The combination of capecitabine and gemcitabine for thymic malignancies has been evaluated in a multicenter phase II study by Palmieri and colleagues.[28] Fifteen patients (12 thymomas and 3 thymic carcinomas) were enrolled and treated with capecitabine at a dose of 650 mg/m^2 orally twice daily from days 1 to 14 and gemcitabine at a dosage of 1000 mg/m^2 IV on days 1 and 8 of a 21-day cycle. The median number of cycles of therapy administered was 6 (range, 3—9). Three patients achieved a CR and an equal number achieved a PR for an overall response rate of 40%. Six patients (40%) had SD for at least 6 cycles. With a median follow-up of 22 months, the median PFS was 11 months (95% CI, 3—17 months). Median survival time had not been reached at the time of publication of results. The estimated 1- and 2-year survival rates were 80% and 67% respectively. Grade 3 toxicities included neutropenia (20%), anemia (13%), thrombocytopenia (13%), nausea and emesis (7%), diarrhea (7%), and hand-foot syndrome (7%); no grade 4 toxicities were observed.

The Japan Clinical Oncology Group Trial, JCOG 9605, was a phase II study of dose-dense weekly chemotherapy in patients with chemotherapy-naïve stage IVA or IVB thymoma.[29] Patients received 9 weeks of treatment with cisplatin 25 mg/m^2 administered from weeks 1 to 9; vincristine 1 mg/m^2 administered on weeks 1, 2, 4, 6, and 8; doxorubicin 40 mg/m^2 administered on weeks 1, 3, 5, 7, and 9; with etoposide 80 mg/m^2 administered on days 1 to 3 of weeks 1, 3, 5, 7, and 9. Granulocyte colony-stimulating factor (G-CSF) was used to prevent neutropenia. Thirty patients were entered on the study and 27 were eligible for analysis to determine clinical response and survival. Eighty- seven percent of patients completed the 9-week regimen as planned. Sixteen of 27 patients achieved a PR for an overall response rate of 59%. Median PFS was reported as 0.79 years (95% CI, 0.52—1.40 years) and median OS was 6.1 years. Survival at 2 and 5 years was 89% and 65% respectively. Major toxicity was myelosuppression. Grade 3/4 toxicity included leucopenia (67%), neutropenia (87%), anemia (83%), and thrombocytopenia (27%). Non-hematological grade 3/4 toxicity included emesis (7%), constipation (7%), and infection (10%).

The objective response rate with this combination was not significantly different from that expected with conventional-dose chemotherapy. The study also failed to meet the expected PFS of 2 years. Hence, dose-dense chemotherapy does not appear to be a promising option for treatment of advanced thymoma.

SUMMARY

Thymoma and thymic carcinoma are chemosensitive tumors. Chemotherapy can be used in the neoadjuvant setting to decrease the size of the primary tumor and resectable metastases to increase the chances of achieving a complete resection. In patients with advanced disease, several different platinum-based chemotherapy combinations have been evaluated as standard front-line therapy. Dose-dense chemotherapy has also been evaluated but not found to offer any significant benefit over standard-dose chemotherapy. In the setting of recurrent disease, single-agent chemotherapy can help in palliating symptoms and improving quality of life. With the advent of targeted therapy, clinical trials are now being conducted to evaluate the safety and efficacy of combinations of standard chemotherapy and biologic agents.

REFERENCES

1. Kondo K, Monden Y. Therapy for thymic epithelial tumors: a clinical study of 1,320 patients from Japan. Ann Thorac Surg 2003;76(3):878—84 [discussion: 884—5].
2. Wright CD, Choi NC, Wain JC, et al. Induction chemoradiotherapy followed by resection for locally advanced Masaoka stage III and IVA thymic tumors. Ann Thorac Surg 2008;85(2):385—9.
3. Ishikawa Y, Matsuguma H, Nakahara R, et al. Multimodality therapy for patients with invasive thymoma disseminated into the pleural cavity: the potential role of extrapleural pneumonectomy. Ann Thorac Surg 2009;88(3):952—7.
4. Yokoi K, Matsuguma H, Nakahara R, et al. Multidisciplinary treatment for advanced invasive thymoma with cisplatin, doxorubicin, and methylprednisolone. J Thorac Oncol 2007;2(1):73—8.
5. Lucchi M, Melfi F, Dini P, et al. Neoadjuvant chemotherapy for stage III and IVA thymomas: a single-institution experience with a long follow-up. J Thorac Oncol 2006;1(4):308—13.
6. Bretti S, Berruti A, Loddo C, et al. Multimodal management of stages III—IVa malignant thymoma. Lung Cancer 2004;44(1):69—77.
7. Shin DM, Walsh GL, Komaki R, et al. A multidisciplinary approach to therapy for unresectable malignant thymoma. Ann Intern Med 1998;129(2):100—4.
8. Venuta F, Rendina EA, Pescarmona EO, et al. Multimodality treatment of thymoma: a prospective study. Ann Thorac Surg 1997;64(6):1585—91 [discussion: 1591—2].
9. Kunitoh H, Tamura T, Shibata T, et al. A phase II trial of dose-dense chemotherapy, followed by surgical resection and/or thoracic radiotherapy, in locally advanced thymoma: report of a Japan clinical oncology group trial (JCOG 9606). Br J Cancer 2010;103(1):6—11.
10. Macchiarini P, Chella A, Ducci F, et al. Neoadjuvant chemotherapy, surgery, and postoperative radiation therapy for invasive thymoma. Cancer 1991;68(4):706—13.
11. Berruti A, Borasio P, Gerbino A, et al. Primary chemotherapy with adriamycin, cisplatin, vincristine and cyclophosphamide in locally advanced thymomas: a single institution experience. Br J Cancer 1999;81(5):841—5.
12. Kim ES, Putnam JB, Komaki R, et al. Phase II study of a multidisciplinary approach with induction chemotherapy, followed by surgical resection, radiation therapy, and consolidation chemotherapy for unresectable malignant thymomas: final report. Lung Cancer 2004;44(3):369—79.
13. Jacot W, Quantin X, Valette S, et al. Multimodality treatment program in invasive thymic epithelial tumor. Am J Clin Oncol 2005;28(1):5—7.
14. Rea F, Sartori F, Loy M, et al. Chemotherapy and operation for invasive thymoma. J Thorac Cardiovasc Surg 1993;106(3):543—9.

15. Bonomi PD, Finkelstein D, Aisner S, et al. EST 2582 phase II trial of cisplatin in metastatic or recurrent thymoma. Am J Clin Oncol 1993;16(4): 342–5.

16. Highley MS, Underhill CR, Parnis FX, et al. Treatment of invasive thymoma with single-agent ifosfamide. J Clin Oncol 1999;17(9):2737–44.

17. Loehrer PJ Sr, Yiannoutsos CT, Dropcho S, et al. A phase II trial of pemetrexed in patients with recurrent thymoma or thymic carcinoma [meeting abstracts 7079]. J Clin Oncol 2006;24(Suppl 18).

18. Umemura S, Segawa Y, Fujiwara K, et al. A case of recurrent metastatic thymoma showing a marked response to paclitaxel monotherapy. Jpn J Clin Oncol 2002;32(7):262–5.

19. Oguri T, Achiwa H, Kato D, et al. Efficacy of docetaxel as a second-line chemotherapy for thymic carcinoma. Chemotherapy 2004;50(6):279–82.

20. Chahinian AP, Bhardwaj S, Meyer RJ, et al. Treatment of invasive or metastatic thymoma: report of eleven cases. Cancer 1981;47(7):1752–61.

21. Loehrer PJ Sr, Kim K, Aisner SC, et al. Cisplatin plus doxorubicin plus cyclophosphamide in metastatic or recurrent thymoma: final results of an intergroup trial. The Eastern Cooperative Oncology Group, Southwest Oncology Group, and Southeastern Cancer Study Group. J Clin Oncol 1994;12(6): 1164–8.

22. Loehrer PJ Sr, Chen M, Kim K, et al. Cisplatin, doxorubicin, and cyclophosphamide plus thoracic radiation therapy for limited-stage unresectable thymoma: an intergroup trial. J Clin Oncol 1997; 15(9):3093–9.

23. Fornasiero A, Daniele O, Ghiotto C, et al. Chemotherapy for invasive thymoma. A 13-year experience. Cancer 1991;68(1):30–3.

24. Giaccone G, Ardizzoni A, Kirkpatrick A, et al. Cisplatin and etoposide combination chemotherapy for locally advanced or metastatic thymoma: a phase II study of the European Organization for Research and Treatment of Cancer. Lung Cancer Cooperative Group. J Clin Oncol 1996;14(3):814–20.

25. Loehrer PJ Sr, Jiroutek M, Aisner S, et al. Combined etoposide, ifosfamide, and cisplatin in the treatment of patients with advanced thymoma and thymic carcinoma: an intergroup trial. Cancer 2001;91(11): 2010–5.

26. Gordon MS, Battiato LA, Gonin R, et al. A phase II trial of subcutaneously administered recombinant human interleukin-2 in patients with relapsed/refractory thymoma. J Immunother Emphasis Tumor Immunol 1995;18(3):179–84.

27. Igawa S, Murakami H, Takahashi T, et al. Efficacy of chemotherapy with carboplatin and paclitaxel for unresectable thymic carcinoma. Lung Cancer 2010;67(2):194–7.

28. Palmieri G, Merola G, Federico P, et al. Preliminary results of phase II study of capecitabine and gemcitabine (CAP-GEM) in patients with metastatic pretreated thymic epithelial tumors (TETs). Ann Oncol 2010;21(6):1168–72.

29. Kunitoh H, Tamura T, Shibata T, et al. A phase-II trial of dose-dense chemotherapy in patients with disseminated thymoma: report of a Japan Clinical Oncology Group trial (JCOG 9605). Br J Cancer 2009;101(9):1549–54.

Targeted Therapies for Thymic Malignancies

Nicolas Girard, MD[a,b,c,*]

KEYWORDS

- Thymoma • Thymic carcinoma
- Epidermal growth factor receptor • Biology • KIT
- Chemotherapy

Thymic malignancies are rare epithelial tumors that may be aggressive and difficult to treat.[1] The current World Health Organization (WHO) classification distinguishes thymomas (types A, AB, B1, B2, B3) and thymic carcinoma.[2] These classes are based on the morphology of epithelial cells (with an increasing degree of atypia from type A to thymic carcinoma), the relative proportion of the nontumoral lymphocytic component (decreasing from types B1 to B3), and resemblance to normal thymic architecture.[2] Beyond histology, the Masaoka and colleagues[3] staging system integrates the degree of invasion and is, together with the completeness of surgical resection, the most significant prognostic factor on overall survival.[4] After surgery, thymomas may present with local and regional progression, whereas thymic carcinomas are highly aggressive tumors with frequent systemic involvement and poor prognosis despite multimodal treatment including radiotherapy and chemotherapy.[5]

Development of cancer results from the accumulation of oncogene activation and tumor suppressor gene inactivation.[6] Large-scale genomic analyses conducted over the past 10 years suggest that cancers may be subdivided in molecular subsets, based on expression, genomic, mutational, and proteomic profiling data. The most complete effort using such "integrated genomic analyses" has been achieved in lung cancer.[7–9] Thousands of genotypic or phenotypic alterations may be identified in tumor cells, but only a few of these are considered to be "driver" alterations that are necessary and sufficient for cancer development and maintenance, a concept also called "oncogene addiction."[10] These single oncogenic pathways may be considered as "Achilles heels" that just need to be systematically identified and exploited using specific targeted agents. This new paradigm offers an optimistic view on new approaches for treating cancer.[11]

Significant efforts have been made to dissect the molecular pathways involved in the carcinogenesis of thymic malignancies.[12,13] Research is hampered by the rarity of the tumor, controversies about histopathologic classification, and the lack of established cell lines and animal models. Insights into the biology of these tumors have been made following anecdotal clinical responses to targeted therapies.[14–18] Here, current knowledge about the molecular data that define molecular subsets and support the use of targeted therapies in thymic tumors is reviewed.

EPIDERMAL GROWTH FACTOR RECEPTOR INHIBITORS

Epidermal Growth Factor Receptor Background

The epidermal growth factor receptor (EGFR) is one of the most studied biomarkers in epithelial cancers.[19] EGFR is overexpressed in 60% to 80% of non–small cell lung cancers (NSCLC), head and neck cancers, and colorectal carcinomas. Since the mid-1990s, small molecule agents—gefitinib (Iressa; AstraZeneca, Macclefields, UK) and

a Department of Respiratory Medicine, Pilot Unit for the Management of Rare Intrathoracic Tumors, Louis Pradel Hospital, 28 Avenue Doyen Lépine, Lyon 69677, France
b Claude Bernard University, UMR 754, 50 Avenue Tony Garnier, Lyon 69007, France
c Radiotherapy Department, Lyon-Sud Hospital, 165 Chemin du Grand Revoyet, F-69495, Pierre-Bénite, France
* Service de Pneumologie, Hôpital Louis Pradel, 28 Avenue Doyen Lépine, 69677 Lyon (Bron) Cedex, France.
E-mail address: nicolas.girard@chu-lyon.fr

Thorac Surg Clin 21 (2011) 115–123
doi:10.1016/j.thorsurg.2010.08.004
1547-4127/11/$ – see front matter © 2011 Elsevier Inc. All rights reserved.

erlotinib (Tarceva; Roche, Basel, Switzerland)—and monoclonal antibodies (cetuximab; Erbitux; Merck, Darmstadt, Germany) have been developed to inhibit wild-type EGFR kinase activity, through competition with ATP to bind the intracellular catalytic domain or inhibition of ligand interaction with the extracellular domain, respectively.[19]

EGFR mutations are the best illustration of the therapeutic relevance of identifying molecular clusters of cancer based on driver genetic alterations. *EGFR* mutations were originally identified in 2004 in tumors responding to EGFR inhibitors.[20] *EGFR* mutations are sufficient for oncogenic transformation in cellular and tetracycline-inducible mouse models.[20,21] In unselected NSCLC tumors, gefitinib failed to produce statistically significant survival benefit versus placebo (5.6 vs 5.1 months; hazard ratio 0.89, $P = .11$).[22] However, when used as first-line treatment in *EGFR*-mutant tumors, gefitinib achieves response rates and progression-free survival incomparably higher than after standard platinum-based doublet chemotherapy (70% vs 30%, and 9.5 vs 6.3 months, respectively).[23] In a routine practice setting, *EGFR* mutation testing is becoming a standard recommendation for the management of patients with lung adenocarcinoma.[24]

Cetuximab has mostly been evaluated in colorectal carcinoma and head and neck carcinoma. Cetuximab significantly increases progression-free survival when compared with standard chemotherapy-based treatment irinotecan as second-line treatment.[25] Combined with standard platin-based doublet in lung cancer, cetuximab prolongs progression-free survival.[26] However, contrary to what was expected given the predictive value of HER2 overexpression on response to trastuzumab (rhuMab-HER2; Herceptin; Roche)

in breast carcinoma, EGFR overexpression by immunohistochemistry in tumor cells was not systematically associated with response to cetuximab.[19] *EGFR* amplification was reported to correlate with response to cetuximab in small series.[27]

KRAS Background

KRAS is a GTPase that is activated by most growth factor transmembrane receptors, including EGFR.[28] Point mutations involving amino acids 12, 13, and 61 lead to impaired GTPase activity, resulting in constitutive activation of downstream signaling cascades. *KRAS* mutations are oncogenic in vivo.[29] *KRAS* mutations are found in 20% to 30% of NSCLC tumors and in 40% to 50% of colorectal carcinoma.[27,30] In NSCLC, *KRAS* mutations are mutually exclusive with *EGFR* mutations.[30] *KRAS* mutations are associated with primary resistance to EGFR inhibitors.[19] Taken together, these data suggest that *KRAS*-mutant tumors represent a specific molecular subset of cancers.[11]

EGFR Expression in Thymic Tumors

Several studies investigated EGFR expression levels in thymic tumors using immunohistochemistry with specific antibodies (**Table 1**).[12,31–37] Overall, EGFR was overexpressed in 33% to 100% of thymic tumors, including 70% of thymomas and 53% of thymic carcinomas. Collectively, there was no strong correlation between EGFR staining and thymic tumor type ($P = .23$, chi-square test) (see **Table 1**). High EGFR staining was significantly associated with stage III–IV tumors ($P = .023$, chi-square test) in 2 studies.[12,34] One study looking at serum EGFR levels also found a correlation with higher stage tumors.[38]

Table 1
Studies reporting EGFR expression by immunohistochemistry in thymic tumors

| | | | Thymoma | | Thymic Carcinoma |
| | | | EGFR Overexpression, | | EGFR Overexpression, |
Author	Method	n	n (%)	n	n (%)
Pescarmona et al 1993[31]	Percentage of cells	15	15 (100%)	NA	NA
Gilhus et al 1995[32]	Intensity	24	24 (100%)	NA	NA
Henley et al 2002[33]	Intensity	31	26 (84%)	6	2 (33%)
Suzuki et al 2006[34]	Percentage of cells	52	22 (42%)	4	4 (100%)
Meister et al 2007[35]	Intensity	17	16 (94%)	3	1 (33%)
Yoh et al 2008[36]	Percentage of cells	21	15 (71%)	17	9 (53%)
Girard et al 2009[12]	Intensity	33	18 (33%)	6	5 (83%)
Aisner et al 2010[37]	Intensity	34	24 (69%)	5	1 (20%)

Abbreviation: NA, not applicable.

EGFR Amplification in Thymic Tumors

EGFR copy number status in thymic tumors was measured in one study including 32 patients.[39] In this study, *EGFR* was significantly amplified in type B3 thymomas. The degree of *EGFR* amplification as measured by fluorescence in situ hybridization correlated with EGFR overexpression by immunohistochemistry in only 30% of cases ($P = .149$), but was higher in stage II–IV versus stage I tumors ($P = .005$).

EGFR Mutations in Thymic Tumors

Following results obtained in lung cancer, several groups investigated whether thymic malignancies harbored *EGFR* mutations.[12,17,34–36,40,41] Thus far, only 3 *EGFR* mutations have been found of a total of 158 tumors collectively analyzed, a frequency of 1.9%. Interestingly, *EGFR* mutations have been found both in thymoma and thymic carcinoma, which are rarely of adenocarcinoma subtype.[2] The mutations were L858R in 2 cases and G863D in 1 case, both occurring in exon 21 encoding the activation loop of the receptor.[36,41] These mutations were previously reported to be associated with response to EGFR inhibitors.[20,42] There was no correlation between EGFR expression and *EGFR* mutational status.

RAS Mutations in Thymic Tumors

Similarly, *RAS* mutations are rare in thymic tumors. In the Memorial Sloan-Kettering Cancer Center study (MSKCC), only 3 (7%) of 45 thymic epithelial tumors harbored such somatic mutations: one was a G12A *KRAS* mutation in a type B2 thymoma, one was a G12 V *KRAS* mutation in a squamous-cell thymic carcinoma, and one was an *HRAS* G13 V in a type A thymoma.[12] Of the 17 thymic tumors previously assessed for *KRAS* status,[17,40,43] no mutation had been identified.

Clinical Relevance

The rarity of *EGFR* activating mutations in thymic tumors explains why responses to EGFR inhibitors have been rarely observed.[40,44] One phase II trial with gefitinib was conducted in chemo-refractory thymic tumors. Among 19 thymomas and 7 thymic carcinomas, partial response and stable disease were observed in 1 and 14 patients, respectively.[40] The recent availability of cetuximab may represent a new avenue for EGFR targeted therapies in thymic tumors. Three observations of heavily pretreated recurrent thymoma exhibiting partial response to cetuximab alone have been reported.[18,45] All tumors harbored strong EGFR expression by immunohistochemistry. A phase II trial is currently evaluating the feasibility of delivering cetuximab in combination with the standard cyclophosphamide, adriamycin, and platin regimen in unresectable thymomas (clinicaltrials. gov ID: NCT01025089).

The recent identification of *HRAS/KRAS* mutations that predict for primary resistance to anti-EGFR–directed therapies[30,46] has to be integrated in trials evaluating cetuximab to avoid "false negative" results. Unfortunately, no effective targeted agents have yet been developed against mutant *KRAS* in the clinic. Overall, *EGFR*- and *KRAS*-mutant tumors represent a very small subset of thymoma.

KIT SIGNALING PATHWAY
KIT Biology Background

KIT (also known as CD117) is a transmembrane growth factor with tyrosine kinase activity whose ligand is the scatter cell factor.[47] The role of KIT in oncogenesis was originally highlighted in gastrointestinal stromal tumors (GISTs), which overexpress KIT in 95% of cases.[48] KIT expression has been associated with activating mutations occurring within exons 9 (extracellular domain), 11 (juxta-membrane domain), 13 (first kinase domain), and 17 (activation loop) of the *KIT* gene.[48] These mutations lead to constitutive activation of the KIT kinase. Imatinib mesylate (Gleevec; Novartis, Basel, Switzerland) is an oral small molecule selective inhibitor of the wild-type KIT kinase that revolutionized the treatment of GISTs by inducing rapid, substantial, and durable tumor responses.[49]

Additional *KIT* mutations, occurring in exons 13, 14, and 17, are identified in GISTs with acquired resistance to imatinib.[50,51] Resistance may be overcome with the use of second-generation inhibitors, such as sunitinib malate (Sutent; Pfizer, New York, NY, USA), a multikinase inhibitor that potently inhibits KIT, platelet-derived growth factor receptor (PDGFR), and all 3 isoforms of the vascular endothelial growth factor receptor (VEGFR-1, VEGFR-2, and VEGFR-3). This suggests that GISTs arise from different types of mutations and may best be treated with different kinase inhibitors.

KIT Expression in Thymic Tumors

After a landmark observation of a KIT-overexpressing *KIT*-mutant thymic carcinoma exhibiting response to imatinib,[14] several studies evaluating the level of expression of KIT in thymic malignancies were reported (**Table 2**).[52–55] All these immunohistochemistry studies used the same anti-KIT rabbit polyclonal antibody from Dako (Carpinteria, CA, USA). Collectively, KIT was reported to be overexpressed in 79 (23%) of

Table 2
Studies reporting KIT expression in thymic tumors

Author	Method	n	Thymoma KIT Overexpression, n (%)	n	Thymic Carcinoma KIT Overexpression, n (%)
Pan et al 2004[52]	RT-PCR	110	0 (0%)	22	19 (86%)
Henley et al 2004[53]	IHC/Intensity	20	1 (5%)	15	12 (80%)
Nakagawa et al 2005[54]	IHC/Intensity	50	2 (1%)	20	16 (80%)
Yoh et al 2008[36]	IHC/Percentage of cells	24	0 (0%)	17	15 (88%)
Tsuchida et al 2008[55]	IHC/Intensity	20	0 (0%)	12	11 (92%)
Girard et al 2009[12]	IHC/Intensity	33	0 (0%)	6	3 (50%)
Aisner et al 2010[37]	IHC/Intensity	34	2 (6%)	5	1 (20%)

Abbreviations: IHC, immunohistochemistry; NA, not applicable; RT-PCR, reverse transcriptase-polymerase chain reaction.

349 thymic tumors, including 5 (2%) of 291 thymomas and 77 (79%) of 97 thymic carcinomas ($P<.001$; chi-square test). Given the significantly highest frequency of KIT expression in thymic carcinoma, some investigators proposed KIT as a diagnostic marker of thymic carcinoma versus thymoma in the setting of a mediastinal tumor.[53] However, the level of expression of KIT also depends on the subtype (squamous cell or non-keratinizing) and the degree of differentiation of the carcinoma.[12]

KIT Mutations in Thymic Tumors

Several groups performed KIT genotyping in thymic malignancies. Collectively, a total of 151 thymic tumors were investigated.[12,14,15,36,49,55–57] Most studies focused on exons reported to frequently harbor mutations in GISTs, ie, exons 9, 11, 13, and 17. Only 5 KIT-mutant tumors (3.3%) harboring 4 different KIT mutations were reported (**Table 3**). All cases were thymic carcinoma tumors.[12,14,36,56] The incidence of KIT mutations was 7% in thymic carcinomas (5 of 70 collectively genotyped). The mutation was in 2 cases a V560 deletion, similar to other mutations described in imatinib-responsive GISTs.[58] Another KIT mutation was an L576P substitution. This mutation was previously reported in GIST and melanoma and was characterized biologically as being sensitive to imatinib and sunitinib.[59] The third mutation was a D820E mutation in exon 17, exhibited by a thymic carcinoma responding to sorafenib tosylate (BAY43-9006; Nexavar; Bayer, West Haven, CT, USA).[56] A KIT mutation at the same nucleotide position (D820Y) was previously reported in imatinib-resistant and sorafenib-sensitive GIST.[60] The fourth KIT mutation was an original H697Y mutation in exon 14,[12] which was not sequenced in other studies. In vitro data suggest that tumors harboring this mutation would be more sensitive to sunitinib than imatinib.[12]

Clinical Relevance

KIT-mutant thymic carcinomas represent a small molecular subset of thymic carcinomas. The clinical relevance of KIT mutations is more limited

Table 3
Growth-inhibitory drug effects in cell lines containing KIT mutations identified in thymic carcinomas

Mutation	Exon	References	Imatinib	Sunitinib	Dasatinib	Nilotinib
V560del	11	12,14	+++	+++	+++	+++
L576P	11	36	+	++	++	+
D820E	17	56	0	0	++	++
H697Y	14	12	+	+++	NE	NE

Abbreviations: 0, Half maximal inhibitory concentration (IC50) >1000 nM, resistance; +, IC50 between 500 and 1000 nM, low sensitivity; ++, IC50 between 100 and 500 nM, mild-sensitivity; +++, IC50 < 100 nM, high-sensitivity; NE, not evaluated.

Data from Girard N, Shen R, Guo T, et al. Comprehensive genomic analysis reveals clinically relevant molecular distinctions between thymic carcinomas and thymomas. Clin Cancer Res 2009;15(22):6790–9; Kuhn E, Wistuba II. Molecular pathology of thymic epithelial neoplasms. Hematol Oncol Clin North Am 2008;22(3):443–55.

than in GIST, as (1) thymic carcinoma harbors *KIT* mutations far less frequently; (2) KIT expression at immunohistochemistry does not represent a good predictor of KIT mutation; and (3) non-pretreated *KIT* mutants are not constantly sensitive to imatinib (see **Table 3**). These findings may explain the absence of responses observed in 2 phase II trials with imatinib, where patients were selected either by histologic type (B3 thymomas and thymic carcinomas)[57] or using KIT staining by immunohistochemistry.[61] Given the rarity of the condition and the existence of molecular platforms for *KIT* genotyping in GIST, our recommendation would be to systematically sequence *KIT* in thymic carcinoma tumors. Ultimately, the use of imatinib should not be recommended, given the higher efficacy of second-generation inhibitors and the results of available clinical trials.[62]

IGF-1R PATHWAY
IGF-1R Biology Background

Insulin-like growth factor 1 receptor (IGF-1R) is a transmembrane receptor that was previously reported to be more frequently overexpressed in squamous cell histology carcinoma tumors. In NSCLC, 70% to 80% of squamous cell carcinoma tumors exhibit high IGF-1R expression levels, when only 25% to 35% of adenocarcinoma tumors do so.[63–65] Although not identified as an oncogenic molecular alteration, IGF-1R activation participates in multiple processes involved in oncogenesis. Recent data from in vitro models suggested that IGF-1R interacts with EGFR through the formation of heterodimers, leading to the trans-phosphorylation of the two receptors,[66] and the activation of common downstream signaling pathways.[67] In NSCLC and sarcoma cell lines sensitive to R1507, a monoclonal antibody against IGF-1R from Roche, IGF-1R phosphorylation was sufficient and required for AKT activation, but minimally affected ERK signaling.[63,68] The growth of cell lines harboring high IGF-1R expression was more readily inhibited after exposure to R1507.[63] IGF-1R activation also participates in resistance to EGFR inhibitors through formation of EGFR/IGF-1R heterodimers, continued activation of the PI3 K-AKT pathway, and inhibition of the pro-apoptotic protein survivin.[67,69] The existence of such mechanisms remains to be investigated in thymic malignancies.

IGF-1R Expression in Thymic Tumors

In a study of 63 thymic malignancies from MSKCC, moderate to high IGF-1R expression by immunohistochemistry was more frequent in thymic carcinomas than in thymomas (86% vs 43%

respectively, $P = .039$).[70] Moderate to high IGF-1R staining was associated with high EGFR staining ($P = .015$ in the whole cohort; $P = .034$ in thymomas). IGF-1R expression level was not a significant prognostic variable on time-to-progression at multivariate analysis (odds ratio 3.07; 95% confidence interval: 0.38–24.59; $P = .291$).

Clinical Relevance

Even if not a prognostic factor, IGF-1R expression may represent a potent predictive marker of response to specific IGF-1R inhibitors. This was observed in NSCLC, for which IGF-1R expression does not influence survival,[63,64] but may be associated with better sensitivity to IGF-1R inhibitors. In a phase II trial including 180 patients with advanced NSCLC, the adjunction of figitumumab (CP751,871; Pfizer) to standard cisplatin-based chemotherapy led to significantly higher response rates (from 32% to 46%).[71]

In thymic malignancies, figitumumab recently showed clinical activity in a patient with refractory thymoma.[72] An ongoing phase II trial evaluates IMC-A12 (ImClone Systems Incorporated, Branchburg, NJ, USA), an anti-IGF-1R antibody, in advanced and refractory thymomas and thymic carcinomas (clinicaltrials.gov ID: NCT00965250).

ANGIOGENESIS INHIBITORS
Angiogenesis Background

Neovascularization is crucial in the development and progression of cancer.[73] Angiogenesis is mandatory for tumors to grow beyond the 1-cm diameter. Numerous pro-angiogenesis factors regulating endothelial cell proliferation have been identified that stimulate vasculature formation, growth of the primary tumor, and migration of tumor cells to the systemic circulation. The most potent pro-angiogenic molecules are those of the VEGFR signaling pathway. VEGFRs are found on the surface of endothelial cells and vascular pericytes, and promote angiogenesis and stimulate cell migration, proliferation, and survival.

Angiogenesis Inhibitors Background

In 2003, VEGF was validated as a clinically relevant target in renal cell carcinoma in a randomized phase II trial comparing the effect of placebo with the anti-VEGF antibody, bevacizumab (rhu-MAb-VEGF; Avastin; Genentech, San Francisco, CA, USA). Bevacizumab significantly prolonged time-to-progression of patients.[74] In NSCLC, addition of bevacizumab to chemotherapy conferred an additional 2-month survival benefit to patients with nonsquamous tumors over those receiving chemotherapy alone.[75] VEGF or VEGFR expression do not appear as predictive markers of response to bevacizumab.

VEGFR Expression in Thymic Tumors

VEGF-A and VEGFR-1 and -2 are expressed in thymomas and thymic carcinomas.[76] Microvessel density and VEGF expression levels have also been shown to correlate with tumor invasion and clinical stage.[77] Patients with thymic carcinomas, not thymoma, also show increased levels of serum VEGF.[78]

Clinical Relevance

Only sparse data are available regarding the use of angiogenesis inhibitors in thymic malignancies. In a phase II trial, bevacizumab was tested in combination with erlotinib in 11 thymomas and 7 thymic carcinomas.[44] No tumor response was observed. In a phase I study with docetaxel and aflibercept, a soluble decoy receptor that binds VEGF-A (VEGF trap), one patient with thymoma experienced partial response.[79] Interestingly, despite the large tumor burden of thymic tumors and the frequent abutment to mediastinal vascular structures, no hemorrhagic side effect has been reported with the use of these drugs.

Multikinase inhibitors may also be of interest in this setting. Beyond the inhibition of KIT, sunitinib and sorafenib also inhibit VEGFR-1, VEGFR-2, and VEGFR-3 at the nano-molar range. The effect of these drugs in thymic carcinoma tumors may then also be related to anti-angiogenic effect.[15,16,56] As sunitinib and sorafenib, motesanib diphosphonate (AMG-706; Amgen, Thousand Oaks, CA, USA) is a specific inhibitor of VEGFR-1, VEGFR-2, and VEGFR-3 that was reported to control for 12 months the growth of a thymic carcinoma tumor refractory to chemotherapy.[80]

OTHER GENETIC ALTERATIONS

Several other molecular targets have been explored in thymic malignancies. HER2, a well-known biomarker that predicts trastuzumab efficacy in breast cancer,[81] is not amplified in thymic tumors, although thymic carcinomas may exhibit HER2 protein expression at immunohistochemistry.[82,83]

The MSKCC integrated genomic analysis included mutational profiling, performed using mass spectrometry—based genotyping. All 45 samples were analyzed for a total of 74 assays, designed to detect known somatic mutations in genes of the EGFR signaling pathway: *PIK3CA*, *AKT1*, *ERBB2*, and *MEK1*.[12] *PTEN* was also analyzed by direct sequencing. No mutation was detected in these genes, which does not support the research use of targeted therapies against these corresponding proteins in thymic tumors.

More recently, several investigators showed that cyclin-dependent kinase (CDK) proteins that control the cell cycle G1-S phase transition, may be altered through p16INK4 loss in thymic tumors, related to gene methylation.[84] A phase II trial with a CDK inhibitor, PHA-848,125AC, is currently ongoing in advanced tumors (Clinicaltrials.gov ID: NCT01011439).

SUMMARY

To conclude, the concept of personalized molecular medicine, which consists of selecting patients for available targeted therapies based on predictive biomarkers, is applicable to rare tumors such as thymomas and thymic carcinomas. Research efforts are currently being conducted to dissect the molecular biology of thymic malignancies. Given the rarity of the tumor, translation of preclinical findings to the clinic may be quick and represents one of the most promising therapeutic approaches for advanced-stage thymic malignancies.

REFERENCES

1. Girard N, Mornex F, Van Houtte P, et al. Thymoma: a focus on current therapeutic management. J Thorac Oncol 2009;4(1):119—26.
2. WHO Histological Classification of Tumours of the Thymus. In: Travis WB, Brambilla A, Muller-Hermelinck HK, et al, editors. World Health Organization classification of tumours. Pathology and genetics of tumours of the lung, pleura, thymus and heart. Lyon (France): IARC Press; 2004. p. 146.
3. Masaoka A, Monden Y, Nakahara K, et al. Follow-up study of thymomas with special reference to their clinical stages. Cancer 1981;48(11):2485—92.
4. Kondo K, Monden Y. Therapy for thymic epithelial tumors: a clinical study of 1,320 patients from Japan. Ann Thorac Surg 2003;76(3):878—84.
5. Eng TY, Fuller CD, Jagirdar J, et al. Thymic carcinoma: state of the art review. Int J Radiat Oncol Biol Phys 2004;59(3):654—64.
6. Hanahan D, Weinberg RA. The hallmarks of cancer. Cell 2000;100(1):57—70.
7. Weir BA, Woo MS, Getz G, et al. Characterizing the cancer genome in lung adenocarcinoma. Nature 2007;450(7171):893—8.
8. Motoi N, Szoke J, Riely GJ, et al. Lung adenocarcinoma: modification of the 2004 WHO mixed subtype to include the major histologic subtype suggests correlations between papillary and micropapillary

adenocarcinoma subtypes, EGFR mutations and gene expression analysis. Am J Surg Pathol 2008; 32(6):810–27.

9. Ding L, Getz G, Wheeler DA, et al. Somatic mutations affect key pathways in lung adenocarcinoma. Nature 2008;455(7216):1069–75.

10. Weinstein IB. Cancer. Addiction to oncogenes—the Achilles heal of cancer. Science 2002;297(5578): 63–4.

11. Pao W, Girard N. New driver mutations in non-small cell lung cancer. Lancet Oncol, in press.

12. Girard N, Shen R, Guo T, et al. Comprehensive genomic analysis reveals clinically relevant molecular distinctions between thymic carcinomas and thymomas. Clin Cancer Res 2009; 15(22):6790–9.

13. Kuhn E, Wistuba II. Molecular pathology of thymic epithelial neoplasms. Hematol Oncol Clin North Am 2008;22(3):443–55.

14. Ströbel P, Hartmann M, Jakob A, et al. Thymic carcinoma with overexpression of mutated KIT and the response to imatinib. N Engl J Med 2004;350(25): 2625–6.

15. Li XF, Chen Q, Huang WX, et al. Response to sorafenib in cisplatin-resistant thymic carcinoma: a case report. Med Oncol 2009;26(2):157–60.

16. Chuah C, Lim TH, Lim AS, et al. Dasatinib induces a response in malignant thymoma. J Clin Oncol 2006;24(34):e56–8.

17. Christodoulou C, Murray S, Dahabreh J, et al. Response of malignant thymoma to erlotinib. Ann Oncol 2008;19(7):1361–2.

18. Farina G, Garassino MC, Gambacorta M, et al. Response of thymoma to cetuximab. Lancet Oncol 2007;8(5):449–50.

19. Ciardiello F, Tortora G. EGFR antagonists in cancer treatment. N Engl J Med 2008;358(11):1160–74.

20. Pao W, Miller V, Zakowski M, et al. EGF receptor gene mutations are common in lung cancers from "never smokers" and are associated with sensitivity of tumors to gefitinib and erlotinib. Proc Natl Acad Sci U S A 2004;101(36):13306–11.

21. Politi K, Zakowski MF, Fan PD, et al. Lung adenocarcinomas induced in mice by mutant EGF receptors found in human lung cancers respond to a tyrosine kinase inhibitor or to down-regulation of the receptors. Genes Dev 2006;20(11):1496–510.

22. Thatcher N, Chang A, Parikh P, et al. Gefitinib plus best supportive care in previously treated patients with refractory advanced non-small-cell lung cancer: results from a randomised, placebo-controlled, multicentre study (Iressa Survival Evaluation in Lung Cancer). Lancet 2005;366(9496): 1527–37.

23. Fukuoka M, Wu Y, Thongprasert S, et al. Biomarker analyses from a phase III, randomized, open-label, first-line study of gefitinib (G) versus carboplatin/

paclitaxel (C/P) in clinically selected patients (pts) with advanced non-small cell lung cancer (NSCLC) in Asia (IPASS) [abstract 8006]. J Clin Oncol 2009;27.

24. Azzoli CG, Baker S Jr, Temin S, et al. American Society of Clinical Oncology clinical practice guideline update on chemotherapy for stage IV non-small-cell lung cancer. J Clin Oncol 2009;27(36):6251–66.

25. Vermorken JB, Mesia R, Rivera F, et al. Platinum-based chemotherapy plus cetuximab in head and neck cancer. N Engl J Med 2008;359(11):1116–27.

26. Pirker R, Pereira JR, Szczesna A, et al. Cetuximab plus chemotherapy in patients with advanced non-small-cell lung cancer (FLEX): an open-label randomised phase III trial. Lancet 2009;373(9674): 1525–31.

27. Laurent-Puig P, Cayre A, Manceau G, et al. Analysis of PTEN, BRAF, and EGFR status in determining benefit from cetuximab therapy in wild-type KRAS metastatic colon cancer. J Clin Oncol 2009;27(35): 5924–30.

28. Bos JL. Ras oncogenes in human cancer: a review. Cancer Res 1989;49(17):4682–9.

29. Fisher GH, Wellen SL, Klimstra D, et al. Induction and apoptotic regression of lung adenocarcinomas by regulation of a K-Ras transgene in the presence and absence of tumor suppressor genes. Genes Dev 2001;15(24):3249–62.

30. Pao W, Wang TY, Riely GJ, et al. KRAS mutations and primary resistance of lung adenocarcinomas to gefitinib or erlotinib. PLoS Med 2005;2(1):e17.

31. Pescarmona E, Pisacane A, Pignatelli E, et al. Expression of epidermal and nerve growth factor receptors in human thymus and thymomas. Histopathology 1993;23(1):39–44.

32. Gilhus NE, Jones M, Turley H, et al. Oncogene proteins and proliferation antigens in thymomas: increased expression of epidermal growth factor receptor and Ki67 antigen. J Clin Pathol 1995; 48(5):447–55.

33. Henley JD, Koukoulis GK, Loehrer PJ Sr. Epidermal growth factor receptor expression in invasive thymoma. J Cancer Res Clin Oncol 2002;128(3): 167–70.

34. Suzuki E, Sasaki H, Kawano O, et al. Expression and mutation statuses of epidermal growth factor receptor in thymic epithelial tumors. Jpn J Clin Oncol 2006;36(6):351–6.

35. Meister M, Schirmacher P, Dienemann H, et al. Mutational status of the epidermal growth factor receptor (EGFR) gene in thymomas and thymic carcinomas. Cancer Lett 2007;248(2):186–91.

36. Yoh K, Nishiwaki Y, Ishii G, et al. Mutational status of EGFR and KIT in thymoma and thymic carcinoma. Lung Cancer 2008;62(3):316–20.

37. Aisner SC, Dahlberg S, Hameed MR, et al. Epidermal growth factor receptor, C-kit, and Her2/neu

immunostaining in advanced or recurrent thymic epithelial neoplasms staged according to the 2004 World Health Organization in patients treated with octreotide and prednisone: an Eastern Cooperative Oncology Group study. J Thorac Oncol 2010;5(6): 885–92.

38. Sasaki H, Yukiue H, Sekimura A, et al. Elevated serum epidermal growth factor receptor level in stage IV thymoma. Surg Today 2004;34(5):477–9.

39. Ionescu DN, Sasatomi E, Cieply K, et al. Protein expression and gene amplification of epidermal growth factor receptor in thymomas. Cancer 2005; 103(3):630–6.

40. Kurup A, Burns M, Dropcho S, et al. Phase II study of gefitinib treatment in advanced thymic malignancies [abstract 7068]. J Clin Oncol 2005;23.

41. Yamaguchi H, Soda H, Kitazaki T, et al. Thymic carcinoma with epidermal growth factor receptor gene mutations. Lung Cancer 2006;52(2):261–2.

42. Chou TY, Chiu CH, Li LH, et al. Mutation in the tyrosine kinase domain of epidermal growth factor receptor is a predictive and prognostic factor for gefitinib treatment in patients with non-small cell lung cancer. Clin Cancer Res 2005;11(10):3750–7.

43. Suzuki M, Chen H, Shigematsu H, et al. Aberrant methylation: common in thymic carcinomas, rare in thymomas. Oncol Rep 2005;14(6):1621–4.

44. Bedano PM, Perkins S, Burns M, et al. A phase II trial of erlotinib plus bevacizumab in patients with recurrent thymoma or thymic carcinoma [abstract 19087]. J Clin Oncol 2008;26.

45. Palmieri G, Marino M, Salvatore M, et al. Cetuximab is an active treatment of metastatic and chemorefractory thymoma. Front Biosci 2007;12:757–61.

46. Qin B, Ariyama H, Baba E, et al. Activated Src and Ras induce gefitinib resistance by activation of signaling pathways downstream of epidermal growth factor receptor in human gallbladder adenocarcinoma cells. Cancer Chemother Pharmacol 2006;58(5):577–84.

47. Zsebo KM, Williams DA, Geissler EN, et al. Stem cell factor is encoded at the Sl locus of the mouse and is the ligand for the c-kit tyrosine kinase receptor. Cell 1990;63(1):213–24.

48. Hirota S, Isozaki K, Moriyama Y, et al. Gain-of-function mutations of c-kit in human gastrointestinal stromal tumors. Science 1998;279(5350):577–80.

49. Demetri GD, von Mehren M, Blanke CD, et al. Efficacy and safety of imatinib mesylate in advanced gastrointestinal stromal tumors. N Engl J Med 2002;347(7):472–80.

50. Heinrich MC, Corless CL, Blanke CD, et al. Molecular correlates of imatinib resistance in gastrointestinal stromal tumors. J Clin Oncol 2006;24(29): 4764–74.

51. Heinrich MC, Maki RG, Corless CL, et al. Primary and secondary kinase genotypes correlate with the biological and clinical activity of sunitinib in imatinib-resistant gastrointestinal stromal tumor. J Clin Oncol 2008;26(33):5352–9.

52. Pan CC, Chen PC, Chiang H.KIT (CD117) is frequently overexpressed in thymic carcinomas but is absent in thymomas. J Pathol 2004;202 (3):375–81.

53. Henley JD, Cummings OW, Loehrer PJ Sr. Tyrosine kinase receptor expression in thymomas. J Cancer Res Clin Oncol 2004;130(4):222–4.

54. Nakagawa K, Matsuno Y, Kunitoh H, et al. Immunohistochemical KIT (CD117) expression in thymic epithelial tumors. Chest 2005;128(1):140–4.

55. Tsuchida M, Umezu H, Hashimoto T, et al. Absence of gene mutations in KIT-positive thymic epithelial tumors. Lung Cancer 2008;62(3):321–5.

56. Bisagni G, Rossi G, Cavazza A, et al. Long lasting response to the multikinase inhibitor bay 43-9006 (Sorafenib) in a heavily pretreated metastatic thymic carcinoma. J Thorac Oncol 2009;4(6): 773–5.

57. Giaccone G, Rajan A, Ruijter R, et al. Imatinib mesylate in patients with WHO B3 thymomas and thymic carcinomas. J Thorac Oncol 2009;4(10):1270–3.

58. Heinrich MC, Corless CL, Demetri GD, et al. Kinase mutations and imatinib response in patients with metastatic gastrointestinal stromal tumor. J Clin Oncol 2003;21(23):4342–9.

59. Antonescu CR, Busam KJ, Francone TD, et al. L576P KIT mutation in anal melanomas correlates with KIT protein expression and is sensitive to specific kinase inhibition. Int J Cancer 2007;121(2): 257–64.

60. Guo T, Agaram NP, Wong GC, et al. Sorafenib inhibits the imatinib-resistant KITT670I gatekeeper mutation in gastrointestinal stromal tumor. Clin Cancer Res 2007;13(16):4874–81.

61. Salter JT, Lewis D, Yiannoutsos C, et al. Imatinib for the treatment of thymic carcinoma [abstract 8116]. J Clin Oncol 2008;26.

62. Ströbel P, Bargou R, Wolff A, et al. Sunitinib in metastatic thymic carcinomas: laboratory findings and initial clinical experience. Br J Cancer 2010;103(2): 196–200.

63. Gong Y, Yao E, Shen R, et al. High expression levels of total IGF-1R and sensitivity of NSCLC cells in vitro to an anti-IGF-1R antibody (R1507). PLoS One 2009; 4(10):e7273.

64. Dziadziuszko R, Merrick DT, Witta SE, et al. Insulin-like growth factor receptor 1 (igf1r) gene copy number is associated with survival in operable non-small-cell lung cancer: a comparison between IGF1R fluorescent in situ hybridization, protein expression, and mRNA expression. J Clin Oncol 2010;28(13):2174–80.

65. Ludovini V, Bellezza G, Pistola L, et al. High coexpression of both insulin-like growth factor receptor-1

(IGFR-1) and epidermal growth factor receptor (EGFR) is associated with shorter disease-free survival in resected non-small-cell lung cancer patients. Ann Oncol 2009;20(5):842–9.

66. Jones HE, Goddard L, Gee JM, et al. Insulin-like growth factor-I receptor signalling and acquired resistance to gefitinib (ZD1839; Iressa) in human breast and prostate cancer cells. Endocr Relat Cancer 2004;11(4):793–814.

67. Morgillo F, Woo JK, Kim ES, et al. Heterodimerization of insulin-like growth factor receptor/epidermal growth factor receptor and induction of survivin expression counteract the antitumor action of erlotinib. Cancer Res 2006;66(20):10100–11.

68. Cao L, Yu Y, Darko I, et al. Addiction to elevated insulin-like growth factor I receptor and initial modulation of the AKT pathway define the responsiveness of rhabdomyosarcoma to the targeting antibody. Cancer Res 2008;68(19):8039–48.

69. Chakravarti A, Loeffler JS, Dyson NJ, et al. Insulin-like growth factor receptor I mediates resistance to anti-epidermal growth factor receptor therapy in primary human glioblastoma cells through continued activation of phosphoinositide 3-kinase signaling. Cancer Res 2002;62(1):200–7.

70. Girard N, Teruya-Feldstein J, Payabyab EC, et al. Insulin-like growth factor-1 receptor expression in thymic malignancies. J Thorac Oncol 2010;5(9): 1439–46.

71. Karp DD, Paz-Ares LG, Blakely LJ, et al. Efficacy of the anti-insulin like growth factor I receptor (IGF-IR) antibody CP-751871 in combination with paclitaxel and carboplatin as first-line treatment for advanced non-small cell lung cancer (NSCLC) [abstract 7506]. J Clin Oncol 2007;25.

72. Haluska P, Shaw H, Batzel GN, et al. Phase I dose escalation study of the anti-IGF-1R monoclonal antibody CP-751,871 in patients with refractory solid tumors [abstract 3586]. J Clin Oncol 2007;25.

73. Folkman J. Angiogenesis: an organizing principle for drug discovery? Nat Rev Drug Discov 2007;6(4):273–86.

74. Yang JC, Haworth L, Sherry RM, et al. A randomized trial of bevacizumab, an anti-vascular endothelial growth factor antibody, for metastatic renal cancer. N Engl J Med 2003;349(5):427–34.

75. Sandler A, Gray R, Perry MC, et al. Paclitaxel-carboplatin alone or with bevacizumab for non-small-cell lung cancer. N Engl J Med 2006;355(24): 2542–50.

76. Cimpean AM, Raica M, Encica S, et al. Immunohistochemical expression of vascular endothelial growth factor A (VEGF), and its receptors (VEGFR1, 2) in normal and pathologic conditions of the human thymus. Ann Anat 2008;190(3):238–45.

77. Tomita M, Matsuzaki Y, Edagawa M, et al. Correlation between tumor angiogenesis and invasiveness in thymic epithelial tumors. J Thorac Cardiovasc Surg 2002;124(3):493–8.

78. Sasaki H, Yukiue H, Kobayashi Y, et al. Elevated serum vascular endothelial growth factor and basic fibroblast growth factor levels in patients with thymic epithelial neoplasms. Surg Today 2001;31(11): 1038–40.

79. Isambert N, Freyer G, Zanetta S, et al. A phase I dose escalation and pharmacokinetic (PK) study of intravenous aflibercept (VEGF trap) plus docetaxel (D) in patients (pts) with advanced solid tumors: preliminary results [abstract 3599]. J Clin Oncol 2008;26.

80. Azad A, Herbertson RA, Pook D, et al. Motesanib diphosphate (AMG 706), an oral angiogenesis inhibitor, demonstrates clinical efficacy in advanced thymoma. Acta Oncol 2009;48(4): 619–21.

81. Piccart-Gebhart MJ, Procter M, Leyland-Jones B, et al. Trastuzumab after adjuvant chemotherapy in HER2-positive breast cancer. N Engl J Med 2005; 353(16):1659–72.

82. Hayashi Y, Ishii N, Obayashi C, et al. Thymoma: tumour type related to expression of epidermal growth factor (EGF), EGF-receptor, p53, v-erb B and ras p21. Virchows Arch 1995;426(1):43–50.

83. Pan CC, Chen PC, Wang LS, et al. Expression of apoptosis-related markers and HER-2/neu in thymic epithelial tumours. Histopathology 2003;43(2): 165–72.

84. Hirabayashi H, Fujii Y, Sakaguchi M, et al. p16INK4, pRB, p53 and cyclin D1 expression and hypermethylation of CDKN2 gene in thymoma and thymic carcinoma. Int J Cancer 1997;73(5):639–44.

Published Guidelines for Management of Thymoma

Yoshitaka Fujii, MD, PhD

KEYWORDS

• Thymoma • Thymic carcinoma • Staging • Classification

In 2009, three papers on the management of thymoma appeared in the literature, citing 58,[1] 69,[2] and 78[3] references and including present day guidelines or recommendations for the treatment of thymoma. There also is a guideline available online compiled by the National Cancer Institute (NCI).[4] This guideline is constantly updated, and this article refers to the April 16, 2010, version. This site lists 10 to 32 references in each of several sections and also contains many useful links. Canadian and British organizations additionally have published online guidelines that are less extensive. The published and online guidelines are physicians' opinions based on case series and phase 2 clinical studies without control groups and thus are at a low evidence level. However, because of its rarity, randomized controlled trials for thymoma (or thymic carcinoma) are extremely difficult to plan. As for treatment options for thymoma, performing a randomized controlled trial is not feasible, because recurrence (7.8%) or death (survival 94.4% at 5 years) is a rare event in thymoma.[5] Thus, careful analysis of the results of case series and phase 2 studies is the only approach allowing to compile the guidelines for thymoma treatment. Ongoing phase 2 studies on thymoma are listed on the Internet.[6] The results of these studies will further help building a consensus for the treatment of thymic epithelial tumors based on better evidence.

This article used the three papers published in 2009[1–3] and the NCI's guideline on the Internet[4] to summarize the consensus on the management of thymoma and thymic carcinoma. The readers are again reminded that all of these are based on the physicians' experience and the results of phase 2 studies and retrospective case series and are prone to future modifications.

HISTOLOGIC CLASSIFICATION AND STAGING OF THYMOMA

The World Health Organization (WHO) histologic classification[7] and Masaoka clinical stage[8] (**Table 1**) are widely used in the literature, in the 2009 published guidelines[1–3] and also in the NCI's guidelines.[4] Thymoma is a neoplasm arising from thymic epithelial cells and is associated with a variable degree of T lymphocyte proliferation. These T lymphocytes are generated de novo within the thymoma from the bone marrow progenitor cells under the influence of the cortical epithelial cell-like function of the thymoma's transformed epithelial cells. In this sense, thymoma is a functional tumor. The WHO classification is based on the morphology of these epithelial cells and the amount of associated T lymphocyte, which is an indicator of the biologic function of the thymoma cells. While thymomas of WHO types A, AB, B1, B2, and B3 all show a certain amount of immature T lymphocytes, thymic carcinomas do not have a measurable number of immature T lymphocytes and are thus undifferentiated. This functional distinction between thymoma and thymic carcinoma is reflected in the 2004 revision of the WHO classification, in which thymic carcinoma is listed as a separate entity from thymoma. Both WHO classification[9,10] and the Masaoka

Department of Surgery II, Nagoya City University Medical School, 1 Kawasumi, Mizuhoku, Nagoya 467-8601, Japan
E-mail address: yosfujii@med.nagoya-cu.ac.jp

Thorac Surg Clin 21 (2011) 125–129
doi:10.1016/j.thorsurg.2010.08.002
1547-4127/11/$ — see front matter © 2011 Elsevier Inc. All rights reserved.

Table 1
Masaoka staging of thymoma

Stage	Description
1	Macroscopically, completely encapsulated; microscopically no capsular invasion
2	Invasion into surrounding fatty tissue, mediastinal pleura, or capsule (determined by pathology[a])
3	Macroscopic invasion into neighboring organs (pericardium, lung, and great vessels)
4a	Pleural or pericardial dissemination
4b	Lymphogenous or hematogenous metastases

[a] Modification by Japanese Association for Research on the Thymus (JART).[13]
Data from Masaoka A, Monden Y, Nakahara K, et al. Follow-up study of thymomas with special reference to their clinical stages. Cancer 1981;48:2485–92.

staging system[8,11] have proved to be strongly correlated with patient survival. These are important factors affecting treatment decision for each patient, and they should be reported in each study. TNM staging of thymoma[12] is not widely accepted, because it is not more useful than the Masaoka system; in fact, lymph node metastases are relatively rare.[5] However, it may be useful for classifying thymic carcinomas that are more frequently associated with lymphatic spread. The NCI guideline does not list thymic neuroendocrine tumors as part of the thymic carcinoma group. This may be reasonable, because neuroendocrine tumors have a better prognosis than thymic carcinoma.[5] The Japanese Association for Research on the Thymus (JART) has made a small modification to the Masaoka staging system in which invasion to the mediastinal pleura (stage 2) is now determined by pathology instead of surgeon's observation.[13] In fact, it is extremely hard for the surgeon to distinguish between benign adhesions to the mediastinal pleura and invasion.

TREATMENT OPTIONS FOR THYMOMA ACCORDING TO THE MASAOKA STAGING SYSTEM
Stage 1 Thymoma

The recommended treatment options are summarized in **Table 2**. A Masaoka stage 1 thymoma is completely resected by surgery, and excellent postoperative survival has been reported after surgery alone. No adjuvant therapy is recommended. Although infrequent, late recurrence is possible, and patients should be followed for more than 10 years. Some thymomas show no histologically definable capsule; in these cases, there is no consensus among pathologists whether these tumors should be included in stage 1 or 2. In patients with myasthenia gravis (MG), total thymectomy is usually performed in the expectation that the procedure will have therapeutic effects on the autoimmune disease. However, in cases without MG, whether a stage 1 thymoma requires total thymectomy for better survival is controversial, and this is the main goal of a clinical study being

Table 2
Recommended treatment for thymoma (stage according to Masaoka)

Stage	Recommended Treatment Option
1	Surgery, no adjuvant therapy[1–4]
2	Surgery; postoperative radiation should be reserved for patients with higher risk* of recurrence,[1,3,4] controversial[2]
3	Surgery; neoadjuvant chemotherapy (radiotherapy) when complete resection does not seem feasible[1,4] Adjuvant radiotherapy[1,4] recommended when incompletely resected[2] Adjuvant chemotherapy, recommended when resection is incomplete[1–4]
4a	Surgery when feasible[1,2,4]; after neoadjuvant chemotherapy[1,2,4] Chemotherapy[1,4] with or without radiation[1,4]
4b	Chemotherapy[1–4]

* Invasion through capsule[1] close margin,[4] WHO B2, B3.[3]

conducted by JART (UMIN000000614). In this trial, clinical stage 1 or 2 thymomas without MG or serum antiacetylcholine receptor antibodies are resected with a wide margin, leaving part of the thymus in the mediastinum. The surgical approach is not clearly defined in the protocol, but most of the cases are resected using video-assisted thoracoscopic surgery (VATS).

With the increased acceptance of low-dose computed tomography (CT) screening for lung cancer, incidental small (<1 cm) thymomas are frequently found. These surely will not affect long-term survival and may even not be resected. However the tumor should be followed on a regular basis, evaluating also the potential effect of thymoma on the onset of MG. However, at least anti-acetylcholine receptor antibodies should be regularly tested in patients with incidental thymomas. Incidental thymomas of larger size are candidates for surgery because of the risk of invasion and dissemination to the thoracic cavity.

Stage 2 Thymoma

The invasion to capsule or mediastinal pleura is rarely diagnosed before surgery; however, stage 2 thymomas are usually completely resectable. Surgery alone confers excellent survival; adding radiation therapy does not offer survival advantages or reduce the rate of local recurrence.[5,14] Adjuvant radiotherapy is not recommended as a routine treatment.[1,4] The recurrence rate of totally resected stage 2 thymoma is 4.1%.[5] Most of these cases present with pleural dissemination. Mediastinal irradiation will surely not prevent pleural dissemination, which is presumably present at time of operation or favored by mediastinal pleural opening. Prophylactic hemithorax radiation is not recommended because of the risk of complications associated with lung irradiation.

Stage 3 Thymoma

Invasion of thymoma to the surrounding organs (pericardium, brachiocephalic vein, superior vena cava, lung, chest wall) is difficult to correctly diagnose at preoperative CT, which tends to overdiagnose. For example, a slight depression of the mainstem pulmonary artery may not be an invasion. In many preoperative stage 3 thymomas, surgery should be considered unless the disease is judged too extensive.

Resectable stage 3 thymoma
If complete resection is feasible, removal of the thymoma en bloc with the invaded organs with a wide negative margin and postoperative

radiation therapy is recommended in all the published guidelines. However, in a recent report of a small series of stage 3 thymoma, survival was not significantly better when adjuvant radiotherapy was added.[15] This needs to be clarified with a larger prospective trial. When the pericardium is involved, postoperative radiation to the heart may result in constrictive pericarditis, which may severely worsen the quality of life of the patient[16] and should be reserved only for selected patients. Neoadjuvant chemotherapy (radiotherapy) is also an option.[1,4] Adjuvant chemotherapy may be considered but not actively recommended for completely resected stage 3 thymomas.[1,4] Adjuvant chemotherapy is recommended for incompletely resected stage 3 thymomas.[1–4]

One guideline[1] posed strong recommendations against bilateral phrenic nerve resection. This is especially true in patients with MG who may need well functioning bilateral phrenic nerves. However, preserving the involved phrenic nerve in these cases does not seem to affect survival.[17] Therefore different considerations should be made in patients with bulbar symptoms or respiratory difficulty caused by MG before the operation.

Unresectable stage 3 thymoma
Unresectable disease is defined as extensive tumor involvement of the trachea, great arteries, or heart[1] or vena cava obstruction, pleural involvement, or pericardial implants.[4] When complete resection cannot be expected at preoperative work-up, chemotherapy with or without radiation therapy is recommended.[1–4] Girard and colleagues[2] and the NCI guideline list surgery or irradiation after induction chemotherapy for inoperable disease,[4] but this option is probably applicable only to a few patients. When surgery is performed, adjuvant radiotherapy is recommended.[2,4] When complete resection is found not possible only at thoracotomy or sternotomy, maximal debulking is recommended,[1] because this procedure seems to improve the survival in the case of thymoma (but not in thymic cancer).[5]

Stage 4A Thymoma (Pleural Dissemination)

Pleural dissemination is not uncommon but is rarely cured. When few pleural implants are incidentally found during surgery, they should be resected, even if a separate surgical approach is required. As many identifiable nodules as possible should be removed with the aim of achieving a macroscopic complete resection. However, this approach may leave inside microscopic tumor nests.

When pleural dissemination is evident preoperatively and is not extensive, surgery with or without neoadjuvant chemotherapy is recommended.[1] The NCI guidelines also list surgery as a potential option after induction chemotherapy.[4] When pleural dissemination is extensive, chemotherapy is recommended.[1,4] Radiation may be applied to focal disease. However, entire hemithorax radiation has been reported to have little impact on the survival in a small group of patients with pleural dissemination.[18] As stated previously, irradiation to the whole pericardium may result in debilitating constrictive pericarditis and should be reserved for selected patients.

A small series of extrapleural pneumonectomy for stage 4A thymoma has been reported.[19] However, because of the high morbidity of the procedure, this indication should be considered conservatively, and no published guideline recommends it.

Stage 4B Thymoma

Chemotherapy is recommended by the published guidelines.[1–4] In cases with isolated local lymph node metastasis, resection of the thymoma and the affected mediastinal lymph nodes followed by adjuvant chemotherapy may be indicated.

Recurrent Thymoma

Three published guideline recommends surgery for recurrent thymoma when feasible.[1,2,4] If unresectable, chemotherapy is recommended.[1,2] The NCI guideline lists the administration of corticosteroid therapy in patients with unresectable thymoma. Steroid pulse therapy may be used for immediate response and show fewer complications.[20] The effect of steroid is probably exerted via the deletion of immature T cells within the tumor and is only temporary. Steroids may be used as a neoadjuvant therapy before attempting complete resection, because they may considerably reduce the tumor volume, in particular if the tumor contains a large number of immature T cells (WHO type AB, B1, or B2).

Patients with MG

Two published guidelines mention the association of MG as a factor that may influence the treatment and survival of patients with thymoma.[2,3] Thymoma is a functional tumor as indicated by the presence of a large number of immature T lymphocytes. As stated before, these T cells are generated de novo by the neoplastic epithelial cells. They are not neoplastic but are not the same as those generated by the normal thymic epithelial cells, because various autoimmune diseases and autoantibodies[21] are associated with thymoma. This indicates that the epithelial cells of thymoma are not fully competent in deleting the autoreactive T cells that are generated within the tumor. As these potentially autoimmune T cells have escaped from the tumor seeding the peripheral lymphoid tissue before the thymoma is resected, complete resection of the primary tumor does not prevent the future onset of MG. Post-thymomectomy MG reported in cases with negative preoperative titer of antiacetylcholine receptor antibody may be an indication of this.[22] This should be taken into account when a very small thymoma is accidentally found on CT in an asymptomatic patient. Also, as the mechanism mentioned previously suggests, the appearance or exacerbation of MG does not necessarily indicate a recurrence of thymoma.[2] When an indication for operation exists for a thymoma, the thymus should be totally resected whenever the thymoma is associated with MG or positive serum antiacetylcholine receptor antibody. Thymomas associated with MG tend to behave less aggressively than those without MG,[2,3,5] probably because the neoplastic epithelial cells are functional and thus are more differentiated than normal ones. Also they tend to be found earlier during assessment of MG patients.

REFERENCES

1. Falkson CB, Bezjak A, Darling G, et al. The management of thymoma: a systematic review and practice guideline. J Thorac Oncol 2009;4:911–9.

2. Girard N, Mornex F, Van Houtte P, et al. Thymoma: a focus on current therapeutic management. J Thorac Oncol 2009;4:119–26.

3. Tomaszek S, Wigle DA, Keshavjee S, et al. Thymomas: review of current clinical practice. Ann Thorac Surg 2009;87:1973–80.

4. National Cancer Institute PDQ Adult Treatment Editorial Board. Thymoma and thymic carcinoma treatment. Health professional version. Available at: http://www.cancer.gov/cancertopics/pdq/treatment/thymoma/healthprofessional. Accessed May, 2010.

5. Kondo K, Monden Y. Therapy for thymic epithelial tumors: a clinical study of 1320 patients from Japan. Ann Thorac Surg 2003;76:878–84.

6. Clinical trials of thymic epithelial tumors. Search for thymoma OR thymic carcinoma'. Available at: http://clinicaltrials.gov/retrieves 52 trials. For studies registered in Japan. Available at: http://www.umin.ac.jp/ctr/index.htm.

7. Travis WD, Brambilla E, Muller-Hermelink HK, et al. Pathology and genetics of tumours of the lung, pleura, thymus, and heart. In: Travis WD, Brambilla E, Muller-Hermelink HK, et al, editors. WHO Classification of tumours. 2nd edition. Lyon (France): IARC Press; 2004. p. 145–97.

8. Masaoka A, Monden Y, Nakahara K, et al. Follow-up study of thymomas with special reference to their clinical stages. Cancer 1981;48:2485–92.

9. Okumura M, Ohta M, Tateyama H, et al. The World Health Organization histologic classification system reflects the oncologic behavior of thymoma—a clinical study of 273 patients. Cancer 2002;94:624–32.

10. Detterbeck FC. Clinical value of the WHO classification system of thymoma. Ann Thorac Surg 2006;81:2328–34.

11. Moore KH, McKenzie PR, Kennedy CW, et al. Thymoma: trends over time. Ann Thorac Surg 2001;72:203–7.

12. Yamakawa Y, Masaoka A, Hashimoto T, et al. A tentative tumor-node-metastasis classification of thymoma. Cancer 1991;68:1984–7.

13. Japanese Association for Research on the Thymus (JART). General rules for study of mediastinal tumors. Tokyo: Kanehara Publishing; 2009.

14. Mangi AA, Wright CD, Allan JS, et al. Adjuvant radiation therapy for stage II thymoma. Ann Thorac Surg 2002;74:1033–7.

15. Mangi AA, Wain JC, Donahue DM, et al. Adjuvant radiation of stage III thymoma: is it necessary? Ann Thorac Surg 2005;79:1834–9.

16. Loire R, Fareh S, Goineau P, et al. Postradiotherapy pericarditis; a clinical and pathological study of 75 cases. Arch Mal Coeur Vaiss 1996;89:1357–62.

17. Yano M, Sasaki H, Moriyama S, et al. Preservation of phrenic nerve involved by stage III thymoma. Ann Thorac Surg 2010;89:1612–9.

18. Yano M, Sasaki H, Yukiue H, et al. Thymoma with dissemination: efficacy of macroscopic total resection of disseminated nodules. World J Surg 2009;33:1425–31.

19. Ishikawa Y, Matsuguma H, Nakahara R, et al. Multimodality therapy for patients with invasive thymoma disseminated into the pleural cavity: the potential role of extrapleural pneumonectomy. Ann Thorac Surg 2009;88:952–7.

20. Kobayashi Y, Fujii Y, Yano M, et al. Preoperative steroid pulse therapy for invasive thymoma: clinical experience and mechanism of action. Cancer 2006;106:1901–7.

21. Romi F, Skeie GO, Aarli JA, et al. Muscle autoantibodies in subgroups of myasthenia gravis patients. J Neurol 2000;247:369–75.

22. Nakajima J, Murakawa T, Fukami T, et al. Postthymectomy myasthenia gravis: relationship with thymoma and antiacetylcholine receptor antibody. Ann Thorac Surg 2008;86:941–5.

The Need for Organization and Collaboration: Establishing a Thymoma Registry

Pascal A. Thomas, MD*

KEYWORDS

- Thymoma • Registry-database • Quality assurance
- Feedback

Thymic epithelial tumors (TETs) are "orphan" diseases, in that they are both rare and neglected. Being rare, their true prevalence or incidence is not well documented. Indeed, the sole national population-based study was published in 2008: the average incidence of all TETs in the Netherlands was 3.2 per million people for the period 1994-2003.[1] The investigators observed that data on slightly less than half of all TETs were collected simultaneously by the Netherlands Cancer Registry, resulting in an incidence of only 1.5 per million for those thymomas considered as malignant in that registry, underlining the complexity and confusion surrounding the histology of these tumors, which remains a debated issue. In the United States, the Surveillance, Epidemiology and End Results (SEER) program collects cancer incidence and survival data and covers approximately a quarter of the US population. Based on the SEER data, an incidence of 1.5 per million for the so-called malignant thymomas was reported for the period 1973-1998.[2]

Because TETs are rare, current knowledge on TETs stems from retrospective cohorts, with reports generally spanning many decades. Furthermore, in addition to the above-mentioned broad diversity of their histology, TETs have an unusual biology and behavior for thoracic malignancies. Local treatments, that is, surgical resection and radiotherapy, are the cornerstone of their management. Even invasive tumors may be associated with a long-lasting fate, marked by iterative surgeries for diagnosis, initial treatment, and recurrence, explaining why 10- or 20-year survival does not necessarily mean cure.[3] This context does not facilitate the setting of prospective controlled trials, the access to biospecimens, or the assessment of systemic treatments or multimodal strategies. Until now, TETs were not of any interest to research and pharmaceutical industries, as well as public health policies.

It is time now for evidence on collaborative efforts to tackle conditions requiring a high concentration of expertise as shown by the growing awareness by patients' associations, health professionals, and decision-makers. To face the diagnostic and therapeutic stakes raised by rare cancers, the French National Cancer Institute has launched in 2010 a call for applications to label a dedicated national expert centers network within the framework of the "Cancer Plan 2009-2013".[4] Scientific societies such as the European Society of Thoracic Surgeons (ESTS) have started with a committed working group. Globalization stimulates coordination of these efforts at an international level to share and disseminate knowledge and best practices, and this concern led to the creation of the International Thymic Malignancy

Department of Thoracic Surgery, University Hospitals of Marseille, University of the Mediterranean, Marseille, France
* Department of Thoracic Surgery, North University Hospital, Chemin des Bourrely, 13015 Marseille, France.
E-mail address: pathomas@ap-hm.fr

Thorac Surg Clin 21 (2011) 131–134
doi:10.1016/j.thorsurg.2010.08.012
1547-4127/11/$ — see front matter © 2011 Elsevier Inc. All rights reserved.

Interest Group in 2009.[5] With the definition of standard operating procedures for handling of surgical specimens and reporting of operative and pathology results, the development of a list of research priorities, and the constitution of tissue banking, the pillar of such a project is the construction of a cooperative registry for medical data collection. This article addresses the expected specifications of this registry.

A DEDICATED REGISTRY

Setting up a dedicated cooperative registry aims at numerous uses, including summarizing the results of the management of a particular disease according to the most meaningful end points; monitoring and improving the quality of care, thereby giving substance to the decision-making process; and serving as a resource for epidemiologic information.[6] At best, it consists of the prospective collection of a predetermined set of clinical, pathologic, and outcome data. On the condition of the control of the most evident sources of errors, it may also be fed retrospectively. The merged information can then be analyzed either as a whole or in parts. Therefore, great care should be taken from the beginning that no key points are missed. Indeed, preparation of a registry requires the initiators to determine the most important questions to be addressed and whether there are enough contributors on the study to achieve those aims. Because epidemiologic issues are to be considered, the registry should also be population-based or should at least sample a representative portion of the population under study.

Recorded Data

A registry dedicated to TETs should include all data on the numerous specific and challenging issues: (1) associated autoimmune and endocrine paraneoplastic disorders; (2) treatment strategies, especially multimodal therapies; (3) rare histologic entities, for example, neuroendocrine entities; (4) surgical approaches used, either minimally invasive or extended surgeries; and (5) consistent pathologic features, such as the histologic subtype and completeness of the resection. Pathology is of pivotal importance. Histologic categorization makes uniform reporting easy and reliable, both in clinical practice and in research. The use of the World Health Organization (WHO) classification for histologic subtyping is only a part of this task. A global checklist to be used in the pathologic evaluation of TETs has thus been generated by the US Association of Directors of Anatomic and Surgical Pathology as an attempt of standardization.[7]

Nevertheless, these efforts of standardization should not restrain information. For instance, this checklist does not address a frequent feature: most thymomas are composite as per the WHO histologic subtypings. It is unclear however, whether the associated prognosis is correlated with the most aggressive subtype or the most preponderant one.

Staging is the end goal of the pretreatment workup. Although the Masaoka staging system has gained widespread acceptance and stood the test of time, one of the first cooperative tasks will nevertheless be the validation of a new staging system for thymic malignancies for standardizing treatment, better predicting the clinical course and prognosis of the disease, and helping to plan the most appropriate treatment strategy on an individual basis. The Masaoka staging system has several relevant limitations. It is not well suited for the staging of carcinomas and neuroendocrine tumors, which are often associated with lymph node and hematogenous metastases, and need more detailed description of these features. It does not provide an appreciable prognostic separation between stages I and II; the definition of stage II is unclear regarding the invasion or crossing of the capsule; stage III is highly heterogeneous and does not segregate the invasion of the great vessels, which has a worse prognostic influence than the invasion of the pericardium or the lung for instance; and stage grouping in locally restricted, locally advanced, and systemic diseases is not well defined.[8] For this reason, all additional information regarding modern imaging methods, including ultrasound-associated thoracic endoscopies, or any attempt at tissue characterization by magnetic resonance imaging, positron emission tomography, or octreotide scanning should be recorded.

Finally, the use of "salvage" medical therapies (eg, biotherapies) or surgical therapies (eg, debulking surgery, extended resections with great-vessel replacement or extrapleural pneumonectomies, surgery for recurrences) should be easily identifiable.

Quality Assurance

Because of this huge amount of information, quality assurance measures for completeness and accuracy of the data should be decided before data collection begins.[9] Data completeness is the extent to which all necessary data that could have been registered have actually been registered. Accuracy of the data is the extent to which the registered items are identical to those in the original source document. There may be many potential sources of errors, and the most frequent ones relate to inaccurate data transcription and programming error in the software used. However, the golden rule is that the more the data are manipulated or transferred, the greater the chance of error. Studies examining this phenomenon have reported that the rates of discrepancies between data fields entered in duplicate in 2 different databases can exceed 25%.[10] The clinical research form (CRF) is an unavoidable medium for data abstraction between the source documents and the database itself. It should be easy to fill, self-explanatory, or accompanied by a glossary for specific headers to give further qualification of that field. Online electronic CRF (e-CRF) presents with multiple advantages in comparison with paper CRF, the most important of which are online real-time monitoring and addressing of queries by data managers. The user interface with the software should be as intuitive as possible. Hierarchic pull-down menus should be used as often as possible, and free-text spaces avoided. The software should incorporate routine utilities for data consistency, alerting on aberrant or contradictory values in some fields. Each patient's file should include some mandatory items to initialize and close the process. Automatic transfer of some fields from the institutional electronic patient's file as source document into the e-CRF contributes to decrease the risks of random errors. In addition, before finalizing the data, the registry should be scrutinized for quality control or monitoring. Routine independent audits are crucial. Ongoing quality controls are more effective than auditing at the time of "data lockout." Regular onsite meetings with all data collectors should alternate with independent external monitoring. These 2 complementary processes allow identification of ongoing systematic errors and avoid their propagation because sources of confusion can be corrected. Periodic data analyses are also necessary to point to discrepancies between sites that may be due to misconception of the CRF and/or the software, which can then be corrected.[11] These aspects raise long-lasting financial issues that will need to be solved while disclosing possible conflicts of interest.

Feedback to Participants

To reflect as close as possible the real-world characteristics of TETs, the registry should be population-based and should involve all the medical surgical teams taking part in the care of these patients. To keep the project alive and gain acceptance of these teams, each participant should receive a continuous feedback. The TET registry should be inspired by 2 examples of existing registries; one is an example of a well-achieved national project (Epithor) and the other typifies a successful cooperative effort at an international level (ISHLT).

Epithor, the French Society of Thoracic and Cardiovascular Surgery (FSTCVS) database,[12] was created in 2002 as a voluntary initiative of general thoracic surgeons. At present, 93 private and public institutions contribute daily to this database, including more than 135,000 procedures recorded until June 2010, which represents more than 70% of all thoracic surgical procedures performed in France annually. Epithor is a government-recognized database, financially supported by the National Cancer Institute for data quality monitoring. Epithor is labeled by the French National Authority for Health, a governmental agency designed to improve the quality of patient care and to guarantee equity within the health care system, as a methodologically correct tool to assess professional surgical practices. Because participating in Epithor is now a part of the required criteria for medical accreditation and unit certification in thoracic surgery in France, all conditions are met for becoming mandatory in the near future. Thoracic surgery units that apply to participate in the French national thoracic database are visited and validated by the coordinator and then sent a confidential code. Variables collected include information about patients' personal characteristics, medical history, surgical procedures, cancer staging, and outcomes. Data are sent through the Internet to the national database; surgeons and patients are anonymous. Each participating center has to implement and download the national database at least every 2 months to avoid becoming temporarily unauthorized to access the database. Participants can check their quality to enter the data by comparing them with national data through a quality score ranging from 0% to 100%. A score exceeding 80% is required to have the local data incorporated in the national database. The exhaustiveness of data collection is also audited IN regular external onsite visitors initiated IN 2010. The national database is updated every 2 months and is downloadable by each participating center, which can then compare its own results with those in the national database in an almost real-time setting. Participants can also use these national data for educational or scientific purposes, provided that they have previously submitted their project to and obtained clearance from the Ethical Committee for Clinical Research of the FSTCVS.

The International Society for Heart and Lung Transplantation (ISHLT) International Registry for Heart and Lung Transplantation[13] was created to provide ongoing, current information on the worldwide thoracic organ transplantation experience.

This registry is currently the only one of its kind and is probably the way to follow at an international level. Every country performing a minimal case-volume of heart/heart-lung/lung transplantation is invited to implement the registry. Data are collected both through individual centers and data sharing arrangement with organ procurement and exchange organizations, such as the United Network for Organ Sharing, Eurotransplant, or the Australia and New Zealand Cardiothoracic Organ Transplant Registry. The collected data, coming now from more than 80 centers worldwide, are made available to ISHLT members and the public via online quarterly data reports and annual data figures, downloadable from the ISHLT Web site. In addition, members may submit own queries to the ISHLT Registry Executive Committee to obtain specific information needed for a research project. The Committee also interfaces with governmental agencies, patients' associations, and international transplant networks.

SUMMARY

The TET Registry project aims at federating an international network to provide a resource to support studies on the epidemiology and clinical management and to monitor some standards of clinical care of TETs. This ambitious project implies the early setting of strong quality assurance measures for completeness, consistency, and accuracy of the data. These measures require a significant and long-term financial support that will also be free of possible sources of conflicts of interests. Data collection for the registry will be done both prospectively and retrospectively through different paths to allow the involvement of as many centers as possible: manual data entry by individual centers via a dedicated Web-based data entry system, electronic download of data from institutional database, and data sharing arrangements with already established databases such as those of the FSTCVS, the ESTS or the Society of Thoracic Surgeons. This project could be a model for other international collaborations, including those for the more frequent thoracic malignancies. Advancements in molecular pathology, genomics, proteomics, and other disciplines may accelerate the current trend toward individual characterization of common cancers into rare subtypes.

REFERENCES

1. de Jong WK, Blaauwgeers JL, Schaapveld M, et al. Thymic epithelial tumours: a population-based study of the incidence, diagnostic procedures and therapy. Eur J Cancer 2008;44:123–30.
2. Engels EA, Pfeiffer RM. Malignant thymoma in the United States: demographic patterns in incidence and associations with subsequent malignancies. Int J Cancer 2003;105:546–51.
3. Venuta F, Anile M, Diso D, et al. Thymoma and thymic carcinoma. Eur J Cardiothorac Surg 2010; 37:13–25.
4. Available at: http://www.e-cancer.fr/plancancer-2009-2013. Accessed September 24, 2010.
5. Detterbeck F, Giaccone G, Loehrer P, et al. International thymic malignancy interest group. J Thorac Oncol 2010;5:1–2.
6. Arts DG, de Keizer NF, Scheffer GJ. Defining and improving data quality in medical registries: a literature review, case study, and generic framework. J Am Med Inform Assoc 2002;9:600–11.
7. Weydert JA, De Young BR, Leslie KO. Recommendations for the reporting of surgically resected thymic epithelial tumors. Hum Pathol 2009;40: 918–23.
8. Bedini AV, Andreani SM, Tavecchio L, et al. Proposal of a novel system for the staging of thymic epithelial tumors. Ann Thorac Surg 2005;80:1994–2001.
9. Pass HI. Medical registries: continued attempts for robust quality data. J Thorac Oncol 2010;5:S198–9.
10. Goldberg SI, Niemierko A, Turchin A. Analysis of data errors in clinical research databases. AMIA Annu Symp Proc 2008;2008:242–6.
11. Rostami R, Nahm M, Pieper CF. What can we learn from a decade of database audits? The Duke Clinical Research Institute experience, 1997–2006. Clin Trials 2009;6:141–50.
12. Available at: http://www.sfctcv.net/pages/epithor.php. Accessed September 24, 2010.
13. Available at: http://www.ishlt.org/registries/heartLung Registry.asp. Accessed September 24, 2010.

Index

Note: Page numbers of article titles are in **boldface** type.

Thorac Surg Clin 21 (2011) 135–138
doi:10.1016/S1547-4127(10)00176-3
1547-4127/11/$ — see front matter © 2011 Elsevier Inc. All rights reserved.

thoracic.theclinics.com

Moving?

Make sure your subscription moves with you!

To notify us of your new address, find your **Clinics Account Number** (located on your mailing label above your name), and contact customer service at:

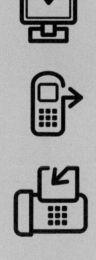

Email: journalscustomerservice-usa@elsevier.com

800-654-2452 (subscribers in the U.S. & Canada)
314-447-8871 (subscribers outside of the U.S. & Canada)

Fax number: 314-447-8029

Elsevier Health Sciences Division
Subscription Customer Service
3251 Riverport Lane
Maryland Heights, MO 63043

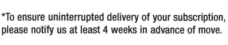

Moving?

Make sure your subscription moves with you!

To notify us of your new address, find your Clinics Account Number (located on your mailing label above your name), and contact customer service at:

Email: journalscustomerservice-usa@elsevier.com

800-654-2452 (subscribers in the U.S. & Canada)
314-447-8871 (subscribers outside of the U.S. & Canada)

Fax number: 314-447-8029

Elsevier Health Sciences Division
Subscription Customer Service
3251 Riverport Lane
Maryland Heights, MO 63043

*To ensure uninterrupted delivery of your subscription, please notify us at least 4 weeks in advance of move.

Printed and bound by CPI Group (UK) Ltd, Croydon, CR0 4YY

03/10/2024

01040351-0017